OXFORD PROFESSIONAL PRACTICE
HANDBOOK OF
Medical Leadership and
Management

T0177746

Published and forthcoming in Oxford Professional Practice

Handbook of Medical Leadership and Management
Edited by Paula Murphy, Peter Lachman, and Bradley Hillier

Handbook of Patient Safety
Edited by Peter Lachman

Handbook of Quality Improvement
Edited by Peter Lachman

OXFORD PROFESSIONAL
PRACTICE HANDBOOK OF

Medical
Leadership and
Management

EDITED BY

Paula Murphy
Consultant Forensic Psychiatrist, East London NHS Foundation
Trust, London, UK

Peter Lachman
Lead Faculty Quality Improvement Programme, Royal College of
Physicians of Ireland, Dublin, Ireland

Bradley Hillier
Consultant Forensic Psychiatrist, West London NHS Trust,
London, UK

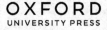

OXFORD
UNIVERSITY PRESS

OXFORD
UNIVERSITY PRESS

Great Clarendon Street, Oxford, OX2 6DP,
United Kingdom

Oxford University Press is a department of the University of Oxford.
It furthers the University's objective of excellence in research, scholarship,
and education by publishing worldwide. Oxford is a registered trade mark of
Oxford University Press in the UK and in certain other countries

© Oxford University Press 2023

The moral rights of the authors have been asserted

First Edition published in 2023

Impression: 1

All rights reserved. No part of this publication may be reproduced, stored in
a retrieval system, or transmitted, in any form or by any means, without the
prior permission in writing of Oxford University Press, or as expressly permitted
by law, by licence or under terms agreed with the appropriate reprographics
rights organization. Enquiries concerning reproduction outside the scope of the
above should be sent to the Rights Department, Oxford University Press, at the
address above

You must not circulate this work in any other form
and you must impose this same condition on any acquirer

Published in the United States of America by Oxford University Press
198 Madison Avenue, New York, NY 10016, United States of America

British Library Cataloguing in Publication Data
Data available

Library of Congress Control Number: 2022946392

ISBN 978–0–19–284900–7

DOI: 10.1093/med/9780192849007.001.0001

Printed in the UK by
Ashford Colour Press Ltd, Gosport, Hampshire

Oxford University Press makes no representation, express or implied, that the
drug dosages in this book are correct. Readers must therefore always check
the product information and clinical procedures with the most up-to-date
published product information and data sheets provided by the manufacturers
and the most recent codes of conduct and safety regulations. The authors and
the publishers do not accept responsibility or legal liability for any errors in the
text or for the misuse or misapplication of material in this work. Except where
otherwise stated, drug dosages and recommendations are for the non-pregnant
adult who is not breast-feeding

Links to third party websites are provided by Oxford in good faith and
for information only. Oxford disclaims any responsibility for the materials
contained in any third party website referenced in this work.

Foreword

As a previous Surgeon General (Head of the UK Defence Medical Services) and now Medical Director of the Faculty of Medical Leadership and Management, I have spent many years in healthcare leadership roles and care passionately about the importance of developing medical leadership capability. I am therefore delighted to have been asked to provide the foreword to the *Oxford Professional Practice Handbook of Medical Leadership and Management*.

Good leadership has a significant role in the success and effectiveness of any team or organization. In terms of healthcare, good medical leadership has a proven positive effect on patient experience and the quality of care provided. It is underpinned by the leader's own values and tenacity. These skills are crucial, and the effect will have a major impact on the contribution of team members and the working environment within the team. This dynamic is also critical to the success of wider collaborations within both organizations and integrated care systems. Leadership is one of those disciplines where there is always something new to learn. Moreover, all doctors require and use the skills of leadership in their clinical practice, so that knowledge and a recognition of a development need should not just be restricted to those in a formal leadership or managerial role.

The seven chapters provide a comprehensive overview to understand the different styles of leadership and the skills that are necessary and must be honed and developed. The handbook rightly differentiates between leadership and managerial attributes but identifies the key managerial competences that are essential to become an effective leader. There are also valuable signposts to further reading at the end of each section.

This handbook is a great introduction for aspiring medical leaders at all career stages and I commend it to you. However, evidence tells us that there is no substitute for leadership learning through practical experience. With this in mind, my plea to all leaders is to create a positive learning environment that encourages healthy debate, a recognition that mistakes/oversights are part of learning, and the importance of building confidence through the team.

GOOD READING!

Dr Paul Evans
Medical Director
Faculty of Medical Leadership and Management
London, United Kingdom

Preface

Leadership is a sometimes mystical yet key component of a clinician's role in health services. Without leadership we cannot deliver safe and effective services. Since the start of the COVID-19 pandemic, the importance of clinical leadership has become even more apparent, in particular to understand and address health inequalities that have manifested along a number of key fault lines.

The *Handbook of Medical Leadership and Management* was conceived at a time when the clinical leadership agenda in the UK was in its infancy, and two of the editors (PM and BH) were trying to understand what leadership in healthcare was, how they could develop the skills, and how to find opportunities to practise them. Some of the knowledge and experience was obtained through mentor–mentee relationships on a leadership programme called 'Prepare to Lead' (initiated by Mr Oliver Warren MD FRCS, and who was its Clinical Director until 2014), which was a forerunner of current leadership initiatives for clinicians. The programme was key in developing supportive networks of like-minded colleagues at a time when healthcare services were undergoing phenomenal changes—as they constantly do! What was felt to be missing at that time was a familiar and easy-reference guide, outlining key concepts and skills with practical examples and signposting, and the idea for this handbook was born.

This handbook has been developed based on a combination of mentor–mentee experiences and learning, combined with our, and others' insights about what we needed to know about why leadership is important, how to be a good leader, and what we need to do to lead effectively. It reflects our understanding of leadership and management in a way we hope is accessible and practical to others. We believe that the things we wanted to know, and which are of vital use to any aspiring clinical leader, are in this handbook. We hope it will help you to develop your understanding of leadership skills, and enable you to integrate these into your clinical practice. We believe that all clinicians at all professional levels are leaders in some form in their own right, and we hope that this handbook will empower readers to confidently lead.

We would like to thank all those who have contributed to this handbook in various ways over the course of time, but in particular Oliver Warren (for setting the scene through 'Prepare to Lead'), our own 'Prepare to Lead' mentors (Peter Lachman and Paul Evans), all the contributing authors listed, as well as the team at Oxford University Press for their continued support.

Dr Bradley Hillier
Dr Paula Murphy
2022

Contents

Contents

Abbreviations

BAME	Black, Asian, and minority ethnic
CMO	contexts, mechanisms, and outcomes
COVID-19	coronavirus disease 2019
CPD	continuing professional development
EBCD	experience-based co-design
GMC	General Medical Council
GP	general practitioner
HFE	human factors and ergonomics
ICHOM	International Consortium for Health Outcomes Measurement
IPU	integrated practice unit
IT	information technology
MRI	magnetic resonance imaging
NHS	National Health Service
P4P	pay for performance
PA	programmed activity
PDP	personal development plan
PDSA	Plan–Do–Study–Act
PREM	patient-reported experience
PROM	patient-reported outcome
RCA	root cause analysis
SLM	service-line management
SMART	Specific, Measurable, Achievable, Realistic, and Time-focused
SPC	statistical process control
SPP	structures, processes, and patterns
WPBA	workplace-based assessment
ZPD	zone of proximal development

Contributors

Dominique Allwood
Chief Medical Officer, UCL
Partners, London, UK
*Chapter 6: Methods and tools to
implement change*

Christopher Bell
Consultant in Community General
and Geriatric Medicine, Croydon
Health Services NHS Trust, London,
UK
*Chapter 4: Leadership for improving
outcomes*

John Brennan
General Practitioner and Quality
Improvement Faculty Royal College
of Physicians of Ireland, Dublin,
Ireland
*Chapter 3: Leading for quality and
safety*

Kezia Echlin
Consultant Cleft and Palate
Surgeon, Birmingham Women's and
Children's Hospital NHS Foundation
Trust, Birmingham, UK
*Chapter 5: Leadership for person-
centred care*

Asanga Fernando
Consultant Liaison (Cancer)
Psychiatrist and Clinical Director of
Simulation and Clinical Skills, King's
College London, London, UK
*Chapter 7: Leadership for clinical
education*

Bradley Hillier
Consultant Forensic Psychiatrist,
West London NHS Trust, London,
UK
*Chapter 1: Introduction to leadership
in healthcare; Chapter 4: Leadership
for improving outcomes; and Chapter
6: Methods and tools to implement
change*

Michael Hobkirk
Consultant Child Adolescent
Psychiatrist, Sussex Partnership
NHS Foundation Trust, Chichester,
UK
*Chapter 2: Management principles for
clinical leaders*

Christopher Holland
Founding Dean, Medical School, and
Consultant, General Adult Intensive
Care, Kent and Medway Medical
School, Canterbury, UK
*Chapter 7: Leadership for clinical
education*

Amrita Kumar
Consultant Radiologist and Clinical
AI Lead, Frimley Health NHS
Foundation Trust, Camberley, and
Chair of AI and Innovation Special
Interest Group, British Institute of
Radiology, London, UK
*Chapter 2: Management principles for
clinical leaders*

Peter Lachman
Lead Faculty Quality Improvement
Programme, Royal College of
Physicians of Ireland, Dublin,
Ireland, Immediate past CEO
International Society for Quality in
Healthcare ISQua,
Dublin, Ireland
*Chapter 2: Management principles for
clinical leaders; Chapter 3: Leading
for quality and safety; Chapter 5:
Leadership for person-centred care;
Chapter 6: Methods and tools to
implement change; and Chapter 7:
Leadership for clinical education*

Alistair Lindsay
Consultant Cardiologist, Royal
Brompton Hospital, London, UK
*Chapter 4: Leadership for improving
outcomes*

Paula Murphy
Consultant Forensic Psychiatrist,
East London NHS Foundation Trust,
London, UK
*Chapter 1: Introduction to leadership
in healthcare; and Chapter 7:
Leadership for clinical education*

Kevin O'Hare
Consultant Histopathologist,
Tallaght Hospital, Dublin, Ireland
*Chapter 3: Leading for quality and
safety*

Lucy Pickard
Consultant Paediatrician, King's
College Hospital NHS Foundation
Trust, London, UK
*Chapter 7: Leadership for clinical
education*

Sean Whyte
Deputy Medical Director and
Consultant Forensic Psychiatrist,
South West London and St
George's Mental Health NHS Trust,
London, UK
*Chapter 5: Leadership for person-
centred care*

Chapter 1

Introduction to leadership in healthcare

Introduction to clinical leadership

Why is clinical leadership important?

A leader is someone whose behaviour, qualities, knowledge, and ideas inspire others to follow them to a common goal. Health leaders strive to improve clinical and quality-of-life indicators and the well-being of the health system.

Clinical training equips clinicians to become experts in the recognition of a patient's symptoms, signs, and interpretation of investigations, to reach a diagnosis and formulate a treatment plan. Many clinicians will work as part of a team to deliver clinical care to a patient and some clinicians will lead, directing the care and identifying a pathway. This form of clinical leadership is very familiar to healthcare professionals and may take many forms (e.g. the consultant who decides and directs the team on what to do versus the consultant who asks different members of the team their opinions and formulates a plan versus the consultant who defers making a decision, pending further information). Clinical leadership is intrinsic to clinicians at all levels of seniority, however, and not just for those who are leading services.

The importance of clinical leadership

Globally, developed economies are operating with an unprecedented demand on healthcare services within a context of resources being stretched. The healthcare environment itself is professionalized, with many individual practitioners having a semi-independent status (e.g. doctors, nurses, and occupational therapists) being regulated by professional bodies beyond the organization within which they work. In addition to the requirement for judicious use of resources, there is a fundamental emphasis on the quality and safety of care. This makes healthcare delivery extremely complex.

In order to meet these demands, while maintaining and improving standards of quality and safety, it has been necessary for healthcare services to fundamentally transform the way in which they function and utilize resources. The traditional view of healthcare treatment (doctors and nurses) and administration (managers) being separate functions has been challenged and found to be lacking. One of the most significant ways that this has occurred has been to look to clinicians to provide leadership for services.

There is good evidence that engagement and harnessing of effective clinical leadership can have a highly beneficial impact on healthcare delivery. Mountford and Webb (2009) provide compelling descriptions from the Kaiser Permanente organization and Veterans' Health Administration in the US, the former conceptualizing the clinical leader as 'healer, leader and partner', and the latter demonstrating dramatic improvements in performance and safety because of clinically informed leadership.

They propose that the changes occurred because clinicians played an integral part in organizational change, were empowered in their professional identity to do so, and were also accountable, whether or not they were in formal management positions. They emphasize the collaborative approach between clinicians and managers to share knowledge and skills in order to make decisions which integrate both clinical and administrative/resourcing demands. In addition, Sarto and Veronesi (2016) carried out a systematic review which identified that healthcare services in which there was a presence of embedded clinical leadership performed better financially, operationally, and for quality of care than those where there was not.

Many developed health systems have recognized that the integration of clinical leadership into healthcare leadership is essential in a modern health service that wants to achieve high-quality care (e.g. Darzi, 2008).

For this to be achieved, it is necessary for clinicians at all levels to develop:

- an understanding of the organizations in which they work
- an appreciation of the complexity of factors from the individual to the systemic level
- an awareness of the constant changes and pressures driving them, as well as their own role and potential in driving changes for this to be effective.

These skills, coupled with a desire to personally develop awareness of leadership qualities, and an ability to communicate a vision of healthcare that empowers patients, staff, and the organization to reach its optimal potential, are the core characteristics of clinical leadership, drawing on a bedrock of clinical knowledge.

The importance of habit

There is increasing recognition that understanding and periodically utilizing leadership skills is necessary, but not sufficient for maximum effectiveness. Using leadership skills for improvement should be a *habit*, permeating behaviour at all levels of the healthcare system (Lucas and Nacer, 2015). Lucas and Nacer bring together five interlocking habits grounded in psychological literature concerning learning, influencing, resilience, creativity, and systems thinking—applied through excellent communication and with the core aims of co-produced health and social care outcome improvement (Box 1.1). Leaders will combine their inherent personal qualities and strengths with development of other skills to lead colleagues, services, and organizations for improved healthcare outcomes, all the time.

Box 1.1 Key habits for leaders

- Developing *systems thinking* to all actions.
- Developing a *learning* environment.
- Being able to *influence* in an empathetic way and to be comfortable with conflict.
- Valuing *creativity* in generating ideas in teams.
- Building *resilience* and being able to take risk.
- Be able to co-produce care and communicate.

Adapted from Lucas and Nacer (2015).

The clinical knowledge to become an effective clinical leader is taught in medical school and developed throughout the medical career. The additional skills relating to clinical leadership are comparatively new and require further experience and effort to develop and practise throughout a medical career.

In this book we aim to equip all clinicians at all levels in healthcare systems with a basis of theoretical knowledge and practical skills to integrate with their own inherent leadership potential, for the benefit of optimal patient care.

References

Darzi, A. (2008). *High Quality Care for All: NHS Next Stage Review Final Report.* [online] GOV.UK. Available at: https://www.gov.uk/government/publications/high-quality-care-for-all-nhs-next-stage-review-final-report (accessed 30/6/2022).

Lucas, B. and Nacer, H. (2015). *The Habits of an Improver: The Health Foundation.* [online] Available at: https://www.health.org.uk/publications/the-habits-of-an-improver (accessed 20/6/2022).

Mountford, J. and Webb, C. (2009). When clinicians lead. *McKinsey Quarterly,* 1 February. Available at: https://www.mckinsey.com/industries/healthcare-systems-and-services/our-insights/when-clinicians-lead (accessed 30/6/2022).

Sarto, F. and Veronesi, G. (2016). Clinical leadership and hospital performance: assessing the evidence base. *BMC Health Services Research,* 16(S2), 169. https://doi:10.1186/s12913-016-1395-5

Further reading

Al-Sawai, A. (2013). Leadership of healthcare professionals: where do we stand? *Oman Medical Journal,* 28(4), 285–287. https://doi:10.5001/omj.2013.79

Health Workforce Australia (2013). *Health LEADS Australia: The Australian Health Leadership Framework.* [online] Available at: https://www.aims.org.au/documents/item/352 (accessed 30/6/2022).

Types of leadership

What are types of leadership?

A leadership type, or style, is the way in which a leader acts or behaves, particularly in relation to their team or colleagues, and can include their manner, outlook, personal characteristics, conduct, and attitude.

Many different leadership styles are described in the literature, with some being considered more effective or desirable than others. Whatever leadership style is adopted, the most important thing for a healthcare leader is to be able to recognize their own style and the appropriateness of that style to the situation, the people, the culture, the context, and the organization.

Why is this important?

Healthcare organizations are highly intrinsic complex systems, working across different specialties and professions, within a managerial matrix, each working towards achieving their own clinical and other outcomes. These different 'groups' within the system operate within their own sub-cultures and can be supporting or opposing of each other. It is therefore vital that leaders within the system can work across the different groups, understanding the complexities, yet ensuring that everyone works towards achieving the common goals of the organization. In understanding the different leadership styles, leaders can adopt and adapt to the best one suited to them and the organization at that moment in time.

What is the theory?

The theory of leadership has evolved over many years. One of the earliest theories was the great man theory, in the nineteenth century. Proponents of this theory believed that leaders were born with inherent characteristics or traits that made them great leaders. This view was eventually challenged, and the focus switched to leaders being described by their pattern of behaviours. This formed the basis of the behavioural theories between the 1940s and the 1980s where leadership styles were described as authoritarian, democratic, or laissez-faire. However, these approaches were criticized for their inability to consider the situation or the context within which the leader worked.

This led to the development of situational and contingency theories between the 1950s and 1980s. Situational theory is based on the premise that the leader must adapt to the style of leadership used according to the situation (i.e. the needs of the organization and the work environment), whereas contingency theory is based on the style of the leader matching the situation—thereby it assumes a more fixed style of leadership.

From the 1970s onwards, interactional leadership theories became more popular with the focus shifting to the relationship between the 'leader' with their 'followers'. In interactional leadership, leaders are seen as either relationship orientated or task orientated.

Other types of leadership styles include transactional leadership, described by Max Weber in 1947. It posits that leaders get what they want from others by using punishment and reward systems and the leader uses a directive style to organize, plan, and set goals. While this is generally deemed to be an insufficient leadership style, there might be situations where it is appropriate and effective. This contrasts with transformational leadership, where the leader works with the team and aims to change the culture of the organization to drive improvements (Box 1.2) (see Types of change, p. 145).

Box 1.2 **Types of leadership**
- Great man—born to lead.
- Behaviour patterns.
- Authoritarian.
- Democratic.
- Laissez-faire.
- Situational or contingency depending on context.
- Interactional between leaders and followers.
- Transactional with reward and punishment.
- Transformational working with the team for change.

Other types of leadership have been described that are not in the scope of this chapter. Nonetheless, some of the key models of effective leadership styles can be applied to healthcare settings. Unsurprisingly, given the complexities within healthcare systems, these models have evolved from situational leadership theory and rely on the leader being able to adapt to different situations and circumstances as appropriate.

Six leadership styles

Daniel Goleman (2000) identified six effective emotionally intelligent leadership styles: commanding, visionary, affiliative, democratic, pacesetting, and coaching. In Table 1.1 these are outlined indicating when they are best employed. All styles should be used to some extent but commanding and pacesetting should be used much less frequently.

Adaptive leadership

In adaptive leadership, the leader encourages people to adapt in order to face challenges and learn new ways of dealing with change. There are four main principles of adaptive leadership, as shown in Box 1.3 (Heifetz, 1994).

Collectivistic leadership

Collectivistic leadership, also known as shared leadership, shifts the emphasis of leadership away from an individual and more towards teams. The traditional vertical model of leadership and leader–follower is replaced by a collective approach and the roles of responsibilities of the leader are shared by everyone. Distributed leadership is a type of collectivistic leadership. Research has found that the best performing organizations in healthcare are ones where there are high staff engagement in decisions.

Distributed leadership

Distributed leadership is a more recently described approach to leadership and is concerned with using a group approach to define the strategy and direction of an organization. It focuses on the distribution of responsibility between everyone in the organization rather than the leader telling the 'followers' what to do. This is illustrated in Fig. 1.1 (Solly, 2018), which depicts distributed leadership and its application in secondary education although the concepts are the same for any organization.

Table 1.1 The six leadership styles

	Commanding	Visionary	Affiliate	Democratic	Pacesetting	Coaching
The leader's modus operandi	Immediate compliance is demanded	People are mobilized towards a vision	Builds emotional bonds and creates harmony	Consensus is forged through participation	High standards for performance are set	People are developed for the future
The style in a phrase	'Do as I say'	'Come with me'	'People come first'	'What do you think?'	'Do at my pace'	'Try this'
Underlying emotional intelligence competencies	Drive to achieve, initiative, self-control	Self-confidence, empathy, change catalyst	Empathy, building relationships, communication	Collaboration, team leadership, communication	Conscientious drive to achieve, initiative	Developing others, empathy, self-awareness
When the style works best	In a crisis, to kick start a turnaround, or with problem employees	When changes require a new vision, or when a clear direction needed	To heal rifts in a team or to motivate people during stressful circumstances	To build buy-in or consensus, or to get input from valuable employees	To get quick results from a highly motivated and competent team	To help an employee improve performances or develop long-term strengths

From Goleman (2000).

Box 1.3 Adaptive leadership

Emotional intelligence
Adaptive leaders build trust by recognizing their own feelings and the feeling of others.

Development
Adaptive leaders are willing to learn and try new things but are also prepared to abandon their ideas if they do not work and will admit if they make mistakes.

Organizational justice
Adaptive leaders are honest and willing to accommodate the views of others so that team members feel valued and respected.

Character
Adaptive leaders are transparent and of good character. They earn the respect of the people that they work with.

Adapted from Heifetz (1994).

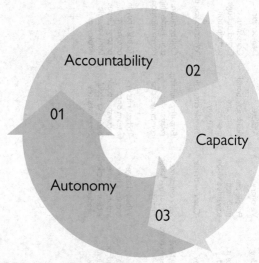

Fig. 1.1 Distributive leadership (Solly, 2018).

Autonomy must be given to the 'leader' within their field of responsibility. If they have autonomy, they are deemed to have accountability for their actions and results. Capacity refers to the 'leader' being provided with the required resources to implement the strategy.

Compassionate leadership

Patient-centred care is increasingly recognized as important for meeting the whole-person needs of the patient (see Leadership for person-centred care, p. 121). This involves providing care that is compassionate, that is, care that that is receptive to the needs and sufferings of others and responds in such a way that it tries to alleviate the problem. In order to provide this type of care across a whole organization, it must be encompassed into the leadership of the organization. This type of leadership is known as compassionate leadership.

Compassionate leadership can be provided in three ways:

- Through the leader showing acts of compassion (e.g. through compassionate words to employees and patients that use words that show understanding of their problems).
- Through compassionate leadership styles (e.g. servant leadership which seeks to develop and engage followers through one-to-one interaction focused on addressing the needs and goals of the followers).
- Implementing structures to enable compassion in a systematic way and nurture a culture of compassion (e.g. collectively noticing suffering and collectively responding to such, collectively allowing a response to grief, staff support programmes, and collective trauma support).

Humble leadership

This is a new leadership model based on humility, vulnerability, and empathy, which form the cornerstone of humble leadership. Its proponents, Peter Schein and Edgar Schein (2018), call for leadership to become more personal so as to ensure more open and trusting communication, thereby allowing for innovation and problem-solving which is collaborative. It moves away from the traditional forms of leadership which are seen as outdated and which are not seen to work effectively in the very complex systems in which healthcare organizations operate. It moves away from the notion of climbing up the ladder and competition between employees.

The premise of humble leadership is that there is an understanding of relationships and group dynamics and that everyone in the organization feels psychologically safe.

Transformational leadership

This type of leadership was described by James MacGregor Burns (1978) in his book *Leadership* and later extended by Bernard M. Bass. In this type of leadership, leaders and followers advance each other to a higher level of morality and motivation. Transformational leaders inspire followers through the strength of their personality and vision and make them change their motivations and perceptions to work towards a common goal. They transform others, developing them to become leaders themselves. Mahatma Gandhi and Nelson Mandela are said to have utilized this type of leadership. This type of leadership is effective in change management and strategic planning.

Participative leadership

This can also be described as democratic leadership and this type of leadership involves including team members in the decision-making process with the leader taking the final decision. The result of this type of leadership is that followers feel more engaged and more willing to work efficiently towards the goals of the organization.

Virtue-based leadership

This type of leadership relies on practising *virtue* ('excellence'). Seven key virtues are identified as trust, compassion, courage, justice, wisdom, temperance, and hope. Respect for others is deeply embedded within it. Proponents of this type of leadership argue that this approach drives excellence and allows for personal growth of individuals, better engagement of people, the development of others, and better performance of the organization. Rather than leading teams through sets of rules, compliance measures, command/control, and extrinsic motivators, virtue-based leadership leads through empowerment, intrinsic motivation, meaning, and virtue-based ethics.

Leadership for careful and kind care

This type of leadership focuses on a return to careful ('attentive concern, solicitude, and error avoidance') and kind ('compassion, kind, gentle') care for patients.

In contrast to this, healthcare has become industrialized, arising from the ever-increasing demands on organizations in the face of decreasing funding and plethora of performance targets to meet. Patients have become commodities, processed through a system as quickly as possible. Care has become transactional. The increased demands on resources and staff mean that staff become too focused on the process and lose sight of the patient. Compassion and empathy for patients are lost and staff become desensitized.

Montori, in his book *Why We Revolt?* (2020), suggests that we need to move away from industrialized healthcare to careful and kind care. This requires leadership as described by Allwood et al. (2022) in Table 1.2.

Table 1.2 Industrialized care versus careful and kind care

Industrial healthcare	Careful and kind care
Hurry	*Elegance*
See more patients in less time	Unhurried conversations through better elimination of other time wasters
Blur	*High definition*
Following guidelines for patients like *this*	Optimal care for *this* patient
Cruelty	*Responsiveness*
Sets of rules, procedures, policies which need to be followed at expense of staff attrition and burnout	Staff well-being prioritized, elimination of policies and procedures that are not helpful
Burden	*Minimally disruptive*
Patients bear the brunt of efficiencies and admin tasks	Care is simple and cocreated by patients

Adapted from Allwood et al. (2022).

Leading for change

Change is an inevitable part of any organization and healthcare organizations in particular need to be able to withstand and adapt to the pressures they face as a result of the ever-changing political, social, economic, technological, and regulatory constraints within which they operate.

There are many models and tools available to assist a leader when implementing change in order to make improvements and these vary depending on what type of change is required (see Chapter 6). One of the most widely accepted models is by John Kotter, who developed an eight-step process for leading change for leaders who want to successfully implement change in any organization (Fig. 1.2).

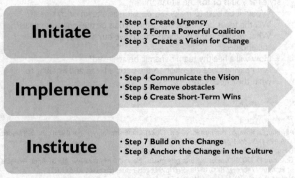

Initiate
• Step 1 Create Urgency
• Step 2 Form a Powerful Coalition
• Step 3 Create a Vision for Change

Implement
• Step 4 Communicate the Vision
• Step 5 Remove obstacles
• Step 6 Create Short-Term Wins

Institute
• Step 7 Build on the Change
• Step 8 Anchor the Change in the Culture

Fig. 1.2 Kotter's eight-step process for leading change (Kotter, 1994).

How does this work in practice?

A leader of an organization might be required to adopt different leadership styles depending on the situation and the context. For example, in a crisis situation such as the COVID-19 pandemic, healthcare leaders had to adopt a commanding style of leadership to redesign services to cope with the huge demand of COVID-19 patients, redeploy staff to acute services, close down non-essential clinics and services, and bring in new COVID-19 protocols and policies. At other times during the crises, however, compassionate leadership was demonstrated by senior leaders through a number of initiatives set up to ease the burden on staff, acknowledge the hard work they were doing, support them, and hear about their experiences. Examples included initiatives such as well-being clinics, free meals, psychological support, tokens of appreciation through small gifts, and regular senior leader (virtual) question and answer sessions for staff.

For some tips for success, see Box 1.4.

Box 1.4 Tips for success

- Be authentic and choose a leadership style that feels comfortable to you.
- Be prepared to experiment—if one leadership style does not get the results you want, try out something else.
- Seek feedback from others.
- Find a mentor who is more experienced and who can offer insights into how they developed as a leader.
- Ask yourself these questions when trying to decide what the right style for you is or for the situation:
  - Would it be best to make this decision as a team or by myself?
  - Will the focus be on the short-term goals or the long-term goals?
  - What would be the best way to achieve buy-in from the stakeholders?
  - How will a healthy team dynamic be achieved?
  - Am I paying close attention to the people I lead and listening to what their needs are?

References

Allwood, D., Koka, A., Armbuster, R., et al. (2022). Leadership for careful and kind care. *BMJ Leader*, 6, 125–129. doi:10.1136/leader-2021-000451

Burns, J.M. (1978). *Leadership*. New York: Harper & Row.

Goleman, D. (2000). Leadership that gets results. *Harvard Business Review*, March–April. Available at: https://hbr.org/2000/03/leadership-that-gets-results (accessed 30/6/2022).

Heifetz, R.A. (1994). *Leadership Without Easy Answers*. London: Belknap Press.

Kotter, J.P. (2012). *Leading Change, With a New Preface by the Author*. Boston, MA: Harvard Business Review Press.

Montori, V. (2020). *Why We Revolt: A Patient Revolution for Careful and Kind Care*. Rochester, MN: Mayo Clinic Press.

Schein, E.H. and Schein, P.A. (2018). *Humble Leadership: The Power of Relationships, Openness, and Trust*. Oakland, CA: Berrett-Koehler.

Solly, B. (2018). *Distributed Leadership Explained*. Sec Ed. Available at: https://www.sec-ed.co.uk/best-practice/distributed-leadership-explained/ (accessed 30/6/2022).

Further reading

De Brún, A., O'Donovan, R., and McAuliffe, E. (2019). Interventions to develop collectivistic leadership in healthcare settings: a systematic review. *BMC Health Services Research*, 19, 72. https://doi.org/10.1186/s12913-019-3883-x

Edwards, L.D., Till, A., and McKimm, J. (2018). Meeting today's healthcare leadership challenges: is compassionate, caring and inclusive leadership the answer? *BMJ leader*, 2(2), 64–67. https://doi:10.1136/leader-2017-000031

Northouse, P.G. (2021). *Leadership: Theory and Practice*, 9th ed. Christchurch, New Zealand: Sage Publications.

Rea, P.J., Stoller, J.K., and Kolp, A. (2017). *Exception to the Rule: The Surprising Science of Character-Based Culture, Engagement, and Performance*. Columbus, OH: McGraw-Hill Education.

Vogus, T.J. and McClelland, L.E. (2020). Actions, style and practices: how leaders ensure compassionate care delivery. *BMJ Leader*, 4(2), 48–52. https://doi:10.1136/leader-2020-000235

Xu, J.-H. (2017). Leadership theory in clinical practice. *Chinese Nursing Research*, 4(4), 155–157. https://doi.org/10.1016/j.cnre.2017.10.001

Leadership and management

Management and leadership have two distinct roles and both are essential to the success of any enterprise.

(Noren and Kindig, 1998)

What is leadership and management?

There is a plethora of definitions of leadership and management and what the differences are between them (Table 1.3) (see Chapter 2).

Kotter (2001) described them as follows:

* *Management*—makes systems of people and technology work well day after day, week after week, year after year.
* *Leadership*—creates the systems that managers manage and changes them in fundamental ways to take advantage of opportunities and to avoid hazard.

Table 1.3 Differences between leaders and managers

Leader	Manager
Strategic helicopter view	Organizes particular part of process
Long-term view	
Focuses on doing the right thing	Short-term view
Sets the vision	Focuses on doing things right
Communicates the vision	Sets the plan
Innovates	Creates stability

Although they are defined separately, the importance of them being considered in conjunction with each other is highlighted by Kotter (2001):

While improving their ability to lead, [organizations] should remember that strong leadership with weak management is no better, and is sometimes actually worse, than the reverse. The real challenge is to combine strong leadership and strong management and use each to balance the other.

Why is this important?

Teams and organizations need a combination of management and leadership to succeed, which requires an environment where innovation and vision are encouraged and supported.

The importance of combining the skills of leadership and management for health practitioners has been recognized globally by various health bodies and institutes, for example, the Institute for Healthcare Improvement (American), General Medical Council (GMC; UK), National Health Service (NHS) Leadership Academy (UK), and Health Workplace Australia (Australian) (see 'Further reading' and 'Signposting'). Empirically based guidance has been developed to help health practitioners encompass these combined skills.

The principles underpinning them are very similar: health practitioners can play vitally important management and leadership roles by influencing improvements in patient care and services. The specific responsibilities include duties related to employment, teaching, training, planning, using resources, raising and acting on concerns, and helping to develop services.

What is the theory?

While the 'function' and 'role' of managers were defined respectively by Henri Fayol (1949) and Henry Mintzberg (1973), with later definitions in broad agreement, the definition of a leader has evolved to encompass a wide range of definitions over the years (see Leadership types, p. 5). Many scholars attempted to describe the differences between the two.

In the 1970s, Abraham Zaleznik first contested the contemporary view of management, which focused on developing ability and power and 'omitted essential leadership elements of inspiration, vision, and human passion—which drive corporate success'. Zaleznik (1977) wrote:

> Managers embrace process, seek stability and control, and instinctively try to resolve problems quickly—sometimes before they fully understand a problem's significance. Leaders, in contrast, tolerate chaos and lack of structure and are willing to delay closure in order to understand the issues more fully.

In 1989, Warren Bennis compiled a record of the differences between leadership and management in his book *On Becoming a Leader*. This included comparisons such as, 'the manager administers; the leader innovates', 'the manager focuses on systems and structure; the leader focuses on people', and 'the manager does things right; the leader does the right thing'. However, the current view has moved away from more critical explanations of management, instead reinforcing the fact that leaders also have a responsibility for safeguarding the healthcare system and resources.

It is now recognized that while leadership and management are separate, they are intrinsically linked and should be considered together to optimize outcomes.

How does this work in practice?

A hospital is a complex system of interconnecting entities required to work collaboratively to produce a common goal.

- This often involves crossing organizational, geographical, professional, technological, political, and economic boundaries.
- It is vital therefore that the senior leaders in the organization, who are often responsible for setting the organization's values, purpose, and goals, work collaboratively with the senior managers who are responsible for ensuring that the delivery of the system is such that it achieves the desired results.
- Both must work seamlessly together, neither one overbearing the other. In reality, the best leaders and the best managers are ones who can tap into both skill-sets interchangeably.

For some tips for success, see Box 1.5.

Box 1.5 Tips for success

The key is to be able to strike the balance between being a leader and being a manager. To do this, ask yourself the following:

- What do you spend most of your time doing? Looking at processes or looking at results? Ultimately, it is the results that matter and as a leader, it is important that you allow your team ways to develop processes in order to achieve the required results.
- What do you talk to the team about? Try to keep the right balance between the processes and the strategy/goal.
- Does the work get done without your intervention? If not, consider directing the team more and trying to find out what is getting in the way.
- Does the team understand the reasons behind what they are doing? It is important that the team understands this to get buy-in and keep them motivated.

Signposting

General Medical Council (2012). *Leadership and Management for All Doctors*. London: General Medical Council. Available at: https://www.gmc-uk.org/ethical-guidance/ethical-guidance-for-doctors/leadership-and-management-for-all-doctors (accessed 30/6/2022).

NHS Leadership Academy (2014). *Clinical Leadership Competency Framework*. London: NHS Leadership Academy. Available at: https://www.leadershipacademy.nhs.uk/wp-content/uploads/2012/11/NHSLeadership-Leadership-Framework-Clinical-Leadership-Competency-Framework-CLCF.pdf (accessed 30/6/2022).

References

Bennis, W.G. (1989). *On Becoming a Leader*. Reading, MA: Addison-Wesley.

Fayol, H. (1949). *General and Industrial Management*. London: Pitman.

Kotter, J. (2001). What leaders really do. *Harvard Business Review*, December. Available at: https://hbr.org/2001/12/what-leaders-really-do (accessed 30/6/2022).

Mintzberg, H. (1989). *Mintzberg on Management: Inside our Strange World of Organizations*. Foster City, CA: Hungry Minds.

Noren, J. and Kindig, D.A. (1998). Physician executive development and education. In: B. Letourneau and W. Curry (eds) *In Search of Physician Leadership*. Chicago, IL: Health Administration Press.

Zaleznik, A. (1977). Managers and leaders: are they different? *Harvard Business Review*, May–June. Available at: https://hbr.org/2004/01/managers-and-leaders-are-they-different (accessed 30/6/2022).

Further reading

Health Workforce Australia (2013). *Health LEADS Australia: The Australian Health Leadership Framework*. [online] Available at: https://www.aims.org.au/documents/item/352 (accessed 30/6/2022).

Swanwick, T. (2019). Leadership and management: what's the difference? *BMJ Leader*, 3(4), 99–100. doi:10.1136/leader-2019-000153

Leadership frameworks

What are leadership frameworks?

Leadership frameworks are evidentially informed conceptual models describing the qualities, skills, and behaviours required to deliver high-quality leadership. They have been developed by various healthcare organizations, both private and public, as well as policy think tanks and academic institutions.

Why are they important?

There is a vast literature of theoretical and experiential evidence arising from decades of research and practice in many different environments (e.g. industrial, commercial, political, and healthcare), from many different disciplines (e.g. sociology, philosophy, and psychology).

Leadership frameworks attempt to bring together this learning, usually categorizing it into more structured models/domains, which can be used from personal to systemic levels. Specific areas where skills and behaviours can be developed by aspiring and current leaders appropriate to the leadership environment are also identified.

What is the theory?

Leadership is pivotal to the sustainability of high-value, high-quality healthcare services and in shaping the culture of organizations, therefore it is crucial that the development of leaders is prioritized to ensure that the right skills and attributes are cultivated. Organizations which have developed leadership programmes and have invested in the development of clinical leaders have shown improved clinical and financial outcomes (Mountford and Webb, 2009).

How does this work in practice?

There are many different frameworks developed for clinical leadership, primarily arising from developed countries and adapted to their healthcare systems. For example, in the UK the NHS Leadership Academy has produced the *Healthcare Leadership Model*, incorporating nine dimensions of leadership behaviour (NHS Leadership Academy, 2013); Health Workforce Australia identifies five important domains where leaders should focus their development and apply their skills for improving healthcare outcomes (Health Workforce Australia, 2013).

In practice, a leadership framework can be used for many different purposes, as shown in Box 1.6.

Using the framework in this way may inform some more specific attributes in a good team leader as seen in Box 1.7.

Box 1.6 Uses of a leadership framework

Leadership frameworks can be used to:
- self-reflect
- identify areas of personal development
- be used to guide a mentor/mentee relationship
- inform a leadership skills assessment in the workplace
- gain feedback from others about one's own leadership skills
- act as the core syllabus for a leadership development programme/be taught didactically through a formal leadership programme
- be used as a guide for those undertaking a clinical improvement project 'on the job'.

Box 1.7 Attributes of a leader

- Set a clear vision and direction.
- Use and develop good communication skills to communicate the vision.
- Ensure objectives are understood by all team members, keeping them updated at all times.
- Agree action plans and achievable deadlines.
- Ensure appropriate time and resources are available for action plans.
- Maintain good political skills by conveying clearly reasoned and rational arguments.
- Identify and correct failures swiftly; identify your own strengths and weaknesses.
- Openly celebrate team successes, advocate for your team at any given opportunity.
- Use political skills to influence the right people at the right time.
- Use clearly reasoned and rational arguments.

Example: the UK NHS Leadership Academy framework

The NHS England Leadership Academy has developed a leadership framework aimed at all clinicians to support their development and utilization of leadership skills in their daily jobs. This evidence-based model is developed on a background of literature review and secondary research to develop a draft model, followed by research through extensive interviews with staff and leaders. The model was finalized in 2013 and is currently used in the English NHS to inform leadership development and to support staff. The framework identifies nine dimensions of leadership as indicated in Fig. 1.3.

In the NHS England leadership framework, the dimensions are graphically arranged with the first dimension Inspiring shared purpose' as the core aspect of clinical leadership, emphasizing its importance.

The framework encourages users to pose questions to themselves relating to each dimension of clinical leadership and to evaluate their own level to which they practise, consistent with the framework. Users are encouraged to be reflective in their answering of each question, rather than just 'yes' or 'no', in order to gain maximum insight into their leadership skills. Helpfully, the framework gives concrete examples of what each domain is

NHS Leadership Academy Nine Dimensions of Leadership

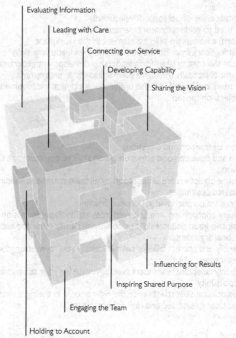

Evaluating Information

Leading with Care

Connecting our Service

Developing Capability

Sharing the Vision

Influencing for Results

Inspiring Shared Purpose

Engaging the Team

Holding to Account

Fig. 1.3 NHS leadership framework (NHS England).
Reproduced under Open Government Licence from the NHS Leadership Academy, Healthcare Leadership Model, 2013.

not, assisting in identification of maladaptive behaviours that may be misinterpreted as leadership qualities.

A key emphasis within the framework is upon personal qualities, particularly self-awareness, self-confidence, self-control, self-knowledge, personal reflection, resilience, and determination. Being willing and able to identify personal strengths and behaviours, both positive and negative, with an openness to developing where necessary, is of crucial importance in becoming an effective clinical leader.

Signposting

The NHS England leadership framework is an accessible and interactive example of a widely recognized leadership framework. It is available at: https://www.leadershipacademy.nhs.uk/resources/healthcare-leadership-model/ (accessed 30/6/2022).

Further reading

Health Workforce Australia (2013). *Health LEADS Australia: The Australian Health Leadership Framework.* [online] Available at: https://www.aims.org.au/documents/item/352 (accessed 30/6/2022).

NHS Leadership Academy (2013). *Towards a New Model of Leadership for the NHS.* London: NHS Leadership Academy. Available at: https://www.leadershipacademy.nhs.uk/wp-content/uploads/2013/05/Towards-a-New-Model-of-Leadership-2013.pdf (accessed 30/6/2022).

Leadership in cultural context

What is leadership in cultural context?

The culture of an organization is determined by the style of leadership employed, which in turn is determined by who provides the leadership.

Why is this important?

White males continue to dominate leadership roles globally, with females and black and ethnic minorities remaining significantly underrepresented. This difference exists despite evidence that diversity in the workplace leads to improvement in healthcare outcomes.

Disparities and discrimination exist in our society and healthcare organizations are no exception. The COVID-19 pandemic has highlighted the disparities that exist in health outcomes according to race, sex/gender, and socioeconomic deprivation. Racism, homophobia/transphobia, misogyny, and disability/religious discrimination represent just some of the biases that exist and while these might not be overt, they exist to some extent or another as unconscious biases. Unconscious biases are 'attitudes or stereotypes that unknowingly alter our perceptions or understanding of our experiences, thereby affecting behaviour interactions and decision-making'.

It is important that organizations acknowledge this because if it is to be addressed then it needs to first be recognized. It is also important because leadership styles between females and minority groups have been found to differ from that of their white male counterparts.

What is the theory?

Research looking at the gender differences of leadership styles have generally found men to be more autocratic and task oriented in their approach (more akin to autocratic and passive leadership styles) whereas women have been found to be more democratic and relationship orientated (more akin to transformational leadership).

Inclusive leadership, that is, leadership that is concerned with treating everyone equally and with respect, has been found to improve performance in organizations. Its focus is on diverse groups and individuals. At an organizational level, inclusive leaders create an organizational culture that embraces diversity between employees, allowing for creativity and innovation. This is seen to benefit the organization, as it leads to improved performance, success, competitiveness, sustainability, and resilience (Edwards et al., 2018).

A theoretical framework on inclusive leadership is provided in Fig. 1.4. Each area includes a list of qualities that characterize a leader.

Another framework which provides a structure to leaders to ensure that they are leading with equity in mind is the *Leading for Equity Framework* by the National Equity Project (2019). The premise of the model is that, rather than leadership being top-down (like traditional leadership), equity leadership is from the inside-out. It bases itself on the idea that 'how we *see* informs how we *engage*, which informs how we *act*'. It provides frameworks that leaders can use to recognize the types of oppression around them; recognize the types of problems in relation to the leadership decision to be made (i.e. problems that are obvious, complex, or complicated) so that the appropriate tool can be used to address the problem; understand

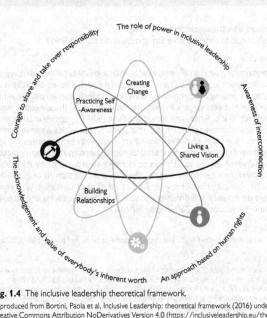

Fig. 1.4 The inclusive leadership theoretical framework.

Reproduced from Bortini, Paola et al, Inclusive Leadership: theoretical framework (2016) under Creative Commons Attribution NoDerivatives Version 4.0 (https://inclusiveleadership.eu/the-inclusive-leadership-handbook-theoretical-framework/).

the current state of the organization's culture; and to design strategies to manage equity problems through experimentation and learning.

Models such as these are useful tools in recognizing and mitigating against unconscious biases in healthcare organizations.

A culture of equity

Advancing Health Equity: Leading Care, Payment, and Systems Transformation is a national programme based at the University of Chicago and in partnership with the Institute for Medicaid Innovation and the Center for Health Care Strategies. It sets out steps to establish a culture of equity:

Identify the problem
- Use the above-mentioned tools to help identify the problem.
- Share data on staff diversity and mix with all staff and leaders.
- Provide opportunities for discussions which might be uncomfortable.
- Get feedback from staff on their experiences.

Take responsibility for improvements
- Prioritize equity in the organization.
- Use standardized techniques to make improvements (quality improvement projects).
- Get senior leaders involved.
- Create equity champions.
- Teach all staff how to recognize bias.

- Ensure that the workforce is diverse.
- Reach out to external diversity groups and establish links.

How does this work in practice?

An organization with an all-male executive board wants to improve diversity within its senior leadership team. It does this through a series of initiatives: it develops a strategy for improving diversity and inclusion across the whole organization; it sets targets to increase the diversity of the executive board by 20% for Black, Asian, and minority ethnic (BAME) representation and a 50/50 male/female split over the next 5 years; it provides an environment for minority groups to thrive, and offers leadership programmes for specific gender/minority groups; it ensures recruitment and selection practices attract diverse applicants; it seeks to increase awareness of all staff within the organization on issues around diversity and inclusion through training and education; it provides regular forums for all staff to engage with senior leaders on equality and diversity issues; it provides mentoring and coaching to minority groups and 360-degree feedback.

Signposting

Inclusive Leadership. [online] Available at: https://inclusiveleadership.eu/ (accessed 30/6/2022).

References

Advancing Health Equity (2012). *Creating a Culture of Equity.* [online] Available at: https://www.sol vingdisparities.org/tools/roadmap/creating-a-culture-of-equity (accessed 30/6/2022).

Edwards, L.D., Till, A., and McKimm, J. (2018). Meeting today's healthcare leadership challenges: is compassionate, caring and inclusive leadership the answer? *BMJ Leader,* 2(2), 64–67. https://doi:10.1136/leader-2017-000031

Further reading

Cuadrado, I., Navas, M., Molero, F., et al. (2012). Gender differences in leadership styles as a function of leader and subordinates' sex and type of organization: gender differences in leadership styles. *Journal of Applied Social Psychology,* 42(12), 3083–3113. https://doi:10.1111/j.1559-1816.2012.00974.x

Inclusive Leadership (2016). *Inclusive Leadership: Theoretical Framework.* [online] Available at: https://inclusiveleadership.eu/the-inclusive-leadership-handbook-theoretical-framework/ (accessed 30/6/2022).

Leading for Equity Framework (2019). *National Equity Project.* [online] Available at: https://www.nationalequityproject.org/framework/leading-for-equity-framework (accessed 30/6/2022).

Livingston, R.W. (2020). How to promote racial equity in the workplace: a five-step plan. *Harvard Business Review,* 98, 64–72.

Marcelin, J.R., Siraj, D.S., Victor, R., et al. (2019). The impact of unconscious bias in healthcare: how to recognize and mitigate it. *Journal of Infectious Diseases,* 220(Suppl 2), S62–S73. http://doi:10.1093/infdis/jiz214

Wilkins, C.H., Friedman, E.C., Churchwell, A.L., et al. (2021). A systems approach to addressing covid-19 health inequities. *NEJM Catalyst,* 2(1). https://doi:10.1056/cat.20.0374

Leadership development: what works?

What is leadership development?

At organization level
This type of leadership development is 'the development of the capacity of groups and organizations for leadership as a shared and collective process'.

At individual level
This type of leadership development, also known as 'leader development', is concerned with leadership programmes aimed at individuals which are delivered by their organization. Individuals learn leadership skills through a variety of ways over a set period of time through a semi-structured programme.

Why is this important?

At organization level
Much of the available evidence on 'leadership development' at organizational level emphasizes the importance of 'collective leadership', which encourages balancing the skill enhancement of the individual with the capacity building of the organization. Collective leadership relies on shared leadership, where a formal hierarchy still exists, but power lies with whoever has the right expertise at that moment in time. Meta-analyses have demonstrated that shared leadership in teams predicts team effectiveness, particularly in healthcare.

Another important aspect of collective leadership is for leadership co-operation, not just within the organization but also across different organizations, as healthcare delivery is dependent on many different agencies working together. Leaders must work together to build an integrated leadership culture.

At individual level
Leadership development of individuals through in-house leadership programmes allows for a variety of leadership skills to be developed through practical, educational, and theoretical methods. These include projects, assignments, role play, lectures, action learning set groups, small/large group sessions, reflective instruments, coaching, and mentoring. Project work is usually aligned with facilitating organizational outcomes thereby being beneficial to both the individual as the leader and to the organization.

What is the theory?

At organization level
Research evidence suggests the value of collective leadership development, particularly at team level. The key to the success of collective leadership development programmes lies in them taking place in-house, rather than remotely, as context is vital—thus emphasizing the importance of organizational development over individual development.

Three key leadership outcomes based on collective leadership have been identified as follows, with leadership development being aimed at each one (Drath et al., 2008):
1. *Direction*: agreement within the collective on goals, aims, and mission.
2. *Alignment*: coordination of knowledge and work in the collective.

3. *Commitment*: the individuals within the collective are willing for their own interests and benefits to be subsumed within the collective interest and benefit.

At individual level

Recent years have seen an increase in studies evaluating medical leadership programmes, which have been mostly from the US (67%) followed by the UK (16%). One systematic review of medical leadership programmes looked at factors associated with outcomes at the clinical and organizational level and found that no particular area of leadership content was associated with improved outcomes whereas project work and/or mentoring was.

How does this work in practice?

An example of this is a healthcare organization which uses collective leadership development to improve its growth and success. It does this by expecting all staff to be responsible for leading the organization. One of the ways it does this is through a leadership development programme which is delivered over 12 days over a period of 12 months and involves staff from all groups and all levels of seniority. Attendees are told that they are responsible for team working, team performance, appraisals, decision-making, and problem-solving. Through the programme, the organizational objectives for development are set out. Staff are asked to take on responsibility for and leading change, after being presented with the trends in the markets and in national and local policies. All staff are valued for the role that they play in the organization.

For some tips for success, see Box 1.8.

> **Box 1.8 Tips for success**
>
> - Promote a partnership relationship between staff and senior management.
> - Support and value frontline staff.
> - Have a strategy for collective leadership.
> - Achieve high levels of staff engagement.
> - Ensure open communication lines between all levels of staff.
> - Ensure leadership development programmes take place in-house rather than remotely.
> - Project work and mentoring is linked with better organizational outcomes.

Reference

Drath, W.H., McCauley, C.D., Palus, C.J., et al. (2008). Direction, alignment, commitment: toward a more integrative ontology of leadership. *Leadership Quarterly*, 19(6), 635–653. doi:10.1016/j.leaqua.2008.09.003

Further reading

Lyons, O., George, R., Galante, J.R., et al. (2021). Evidence-based medical leadership development: a systematic review. *BMJ Leader*, 5(3), 206–213. doi:10.1136/leader-2020-000360

McKimm, J., Hickford, D., Lees, P., et al. (2019). Evaluating the impact of a national clinical leadership fellow scheme. *BMJ Leader*, 3(2), 37–42. doi:10.1136/leader-2019-000135

Seidman, G., Pascal, L., and McDonough, J. (2020). What benefits do healthcare organisations receive from leadership and management development programmes? A systematic review of the evidence. *BMJ Leader*, 4(1), 21–36. doi:10.1136/leader-2019-000141

West, M., Armit, K., Loewenthal, L., et al. (2015). *Leadership and Leadership Development in Health Care*. [online] Faculty of Medical Leadership and Management, The King's Fund, and the Centre for Creative Leadership. Available at: https://www.kingsfund.org.uk/publications/leadership-and-leadership-development-health-care (accessed 30/6/2022).

West, M., Eckert, R., Steward, K., et al. (2014). *Developing Collective Leadership for Health Care*. [online] The Kings Fund. Available at: https://www.kingsfund.org.uk/sites/default/files/field/field_publication_file/developing-collective-leadership-kingsfund-may14.pdf (accessed 30/6/2022).

Leadership and practitioner well-being

What is leadership and practitioner well-being and why is it important?

The increased understanding of associations between practitioner health and well-being (especially mental health), staff morale, recruitment and retention, patient safety, and quality of care have an overarching relevance to all areas of leadership and practice.

The well-being of the workforce is one of the most valuable assets for any medical leader, as well as their own personal health and well-being. There has been increasing interest in this area following recognition that healthcare professionals have higher rates of depression, substance use, and suicide as compared to the general population.

The COVID-19 pandemic has been associated with extreme pressures, increased reports of burnout among practitioners, and moral injury when difficult decisions regarding provision of care have needed to be made. While there was an appreciation of the importance of practitioner health prior to this, the pandemic has brought the issue into sharp focus and accelerated developments in this area, with the World Health Organization prioritizing health worker's safety for World Patient Safety Day in 2020.

It is important that leaders understand the ways to foster an approach within their organizations that allows for the provision of support to prevent health problems from escalating initially, while also developing a professional environment where those with more evident problems can access the correct care. Appropriate integration of an ethos to support practitioner health both improves the well-being in general but also can improve recruitment and retention and, as importantly, have an impact on patient safety and quality of care.

In this topic, we will focus on burnout and its manifestations among practitioners (in particular, mental health), the impact of this on patient safety and organizational well-being, and the ways in which leaders and organizations can anticipate and respond to these, including a framework developed in Australia, and one in the US.

Work-related stress and burnout

Work-related stress can be defined as 'the adverse reaction people have to excessive pressures or other types of demand placed on them'. Surveys such as the Annual UK Labour Force Survey consistently report the highest rates of stress, depression, and anxiety in healthcare workforces than any other sector. Unchecked, such stressors can contribute to the syndrome of 'burnout', described by Maslach et al. (2001) as a prolonged response to chronic emotional and interpersonal stressors on the job; this was pithily described as:

> What started out as important, meaningful, and challenging work becomes unpleasant, unfulfilling, and meaningless. Energy turns into exhaustion, involvement turns into cynicism, and efficacy turns into ineffectiveness.

The causes of burnout are complex, but surveys internationally of healthcare professionals have identified several (relatively unsurprising) factors, including increasing workload, time pressures, reducing pay, chaotic work environments, completing more and unproductive bureaucratic tasks, and feeling like 'cogs in a system'.

In the US, a study commissioned by the American Association of Medical Colleges indicated that the impact of burnout and mental health difficulties is projected to result in a worsened shortage of physicians over coming decades, resulting from professionals leaving medicine mid-career and cutting back hours. In the context of workforce shortages, this can lead to a vicious cycle, whereby doctors become ill from stress/exhaustion, leading to sickness leave, changes in working practice, or leaving the profession. Consequently, there are fewer doctors to fulfil the remaining tasks, and they then have to work harder, thereby increasing their levels of stress and risk of becoming ill. According to the GMC's *Adapting, Coping, Compromising* research in 2018, up to 12% of practitioners took leave in the previous year owing to stress. In addition, owing to such pressures there is a tendency to prioritize immediate and urgent tasks, which can impact the ability to participate in team building and continuing professional development (CPD) activities.

There is evidence that during the COVID-19 pandemic, burnout rates have increased to very high levels as compared to previous years. Monitoring by the GMC through National Training Surveys, involving around 63,000 practitioners, has demonstrated that using the Copenhagen Burnout Inventory, one-third of trainees said they felt burnt out to a high/very high degree because of their work, compared to around one-quarter in previous years. This increase was also mirrored by 25% of secondary care trainers reporting the same levels of burnout, and 22% of general practitioners (GPs).

Rates of mental health problems among practitioners

Practitioners are at an increased risk of mental health problems as compared to the general population. An extensive report from the Society of Occupational Medicine (Kinman and Teoh, 2018) demonstrated that there was a prevalence of common mental disorders among UK practitioners of around 30% in general, although since these findings arose mainly from self-report questionnaires, they are thought likely to be underestimates, and may also demonstrate the 'healthy worker' effect, with practitioners who are too unwell likely to already be on sick leave or having left working in healthcare. A survey of GPs suggested that up to 95% of respondents were likely to be suffering from a minor psychiatric disorder.

Depression has been shown to have increased rates in practitioners, with one meta-analysis showing increased depressive symptoms developing throughout years of training, from 15.8% in the first year to between 20% and 40%. Substance use is also recognized to be increased in healthcare professionals, with a National Health Practitioner Health Programme describing up to 15% of their caseload as being comprised of individuals using alcohol and/or substances harmfully (Gerada, 2018). These have also been comprehensively reviewed by Harvey et al. (2021) in a recent *Lancet* review.

Of particular concern is the higher rates of suicide in practitioners. Gerada (2018) described that thoughts of suicide are significantly higher compared to the general population and other professionals (24.8% vs 13.3% vs 12.8%, respectively), and the relative suicide risk was 1.1–3.4 for men and 2.5–5.7 for women. Additional characteristics which may increase the risk among practitioners include awareness of toxicological issues, access to lethal medications, and potential to turn their own expertise to lethal use. Accessing timely intervention is a significant factor which can hinder suicide prevention in healthcare practitioners, as can patient safety-related consequences of ill health leading to investigation by professional regulators.

Barriers in practitioners accessing healthcare

It has been suggested that acculturation is especially important regarding practitioners' health access, and which can be the most difficult for an individual to address (Kay et al., 2008). For many practitioners, acculturation begins in medical school, and propagates stigma concerning illness. This stigma is further compounded when the manifestation of health problems is through mental illness and/or addiction, with fears about the impact on future career prospects and associated worries about fitness to practise being synergistic. Practitioners also experience barriers in accessing healthcare through a variety of mechanisms as detailed in Box 1.9.

Box 1.9 Barriers to practitioners accessing healthcare

- 'Embarrassment' (e.g. feeling that their problem was trivial and should not impose on another practitioner's time).
- Lack of time.
- Fears about confidentiality.
- Shame.
- Lack of structural support within healthcare systems.
- Preference to seek 'informal' solutions, such as speaking with colleague, or self-medication.
- Cultural aspects of medicine whereby a sense of 'pressure to be healthy' prevails from within the medical community and from colleagues.

Impact on patient safety and experience

There is evidence that burnout and associated health problems of practitioners are associated with problems in safety-related quality of care. Hall et al. (2016) carried out a systematic review demonstrating that poor well-being (characterized by depression, anxiety, poor quality of life and stress, and high levels of burnout) were significantly associated with more self-reported errors, and objective measures of error. These may be mediated through distracted behaviour, poor decision-making, impaired attention, reduced quality of communication with patients and peers, and feeling less empathy. Conversely, good staff health has been associated with reduced methicillin-resistance *Staphylococcus aureus* (MRSA) rates, lower standardized mortality figures, improved patient experience of care and patient satisfaction, lower rates of sickness absence and use of agency staff, and improved productivity.

Firth-Cozens (2001) described a model whereby the feedback of occupational and organizational stressors coupled with individual differences can impact the well-being of doctors, and thus ultimately contribute to poor patient care, as shown in Fig. 1.5. In addition, interventions that can occur to address these are described (see below).

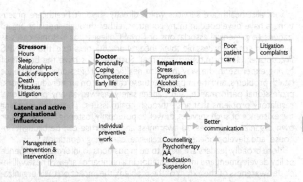

Fig. 1.5 A systems approach to the causes of poor patient care.

Reproduced with permission from Firth-Cozens, J. (2001). Cultures for improving patient safety through learning: the role of teamwork. *Quality in Health Care: QHC*, 10(Suppl 2), ii26–ii31.

Approaches to improving practitioner well-being

Leaders can impact the well-being of the workforce in several powerful ways, including at the level of their own behaviour, within their organization, and through raising awareness and influencing policy on a regional, national, and international level.

Perhaps the single most important aspect of improving practitioner and workforce well-being is that a leader can influence is fostering an organization's culture to be one of openness about work-related pressure and mental health, associated with good staff management, fairness, and supportiveness. Approaches that have been introduced to many healthcare organizations include the provision of robust occupational health services which include access to confidential support services not requiring line management authorization or awareness. Increased training of staff in positions of people management to recognize when work-related performance issues may be a manifestation of burnout and/or health problems can also be promoted.

Within some healthcare organizations, chief executives have championed the introduction of Schwartz Rounds™. Unlike traditional medical 'grand rounds', they provide a monthly reflective space where all staff (clinical and non-clinical) come together to discuss the emotional and social aspects of working in healthcare. They have been developed in numerous healthcare systems in the US, Canada, the UK, Ireland, Australia, and New Zealand. These reflective spaces provide a focus on the experiences, thoughts, and feelings experienced by caregivers using actual patient cases. Following a brief presentation regarding a patient or topic, caregivers in attendance are invited to share their own perspectives and broader related issues. Of note, they are not presentations to determine aspects of that patient's care. In a national evaluation in the UK, there was a reported 50% reduction in psychological distress in regular attenders (from 27% to 34%) as compared to non-attenders.

Specialist healthcare services which directly support healthcare practitioners have developed in many countries, either through specialty organizations (e.g. medical associations or Royal Colleges), or in some cases as a national service accessible to all medical practitioners (e.g. the UK NHS Practitioner Health (n.d.) programme). Such services have the benefit of having expertise in the way in which healthcare professionals experience health problems, and the impact that these can have on an individual's work, professional performance, and patient safety, as well as any professional regulatory problems that arise through health issues. Through supporting the existence of such services, as well as potentially fostering links with your own organization, increased awareness and expertise can be brought 'in-house' and develop pockets of excellence, enhancing reputation.

More broadly, leaders are likely to be in positions to inform and influence policy development and implementation in a number of areas. These will include awareness of the extent of the problem, the impact on their organizations in terms of cost, performance, and safety, and how this interacts with broader employment and in particular professional regulatory implications for practitioners. Although outside the scope of this handbook, the multiple duties and allegiances to their employer and also their professional regulator which a healthcare practitioner balances can become disrupted in cases of ill health; for most healthcare practitioners, whose professional role and identity can be closely linked, even a referral to the regulator can be a deeply traumatic and risk-increasing situation. The increasing awareness of the increased risk for healthcare professionals to experience problems with their health (including addiction problems), as well as the presence of advocates in leadership positions to provide a de-stigmatizing voice has, and will continue to be, an important mechanism through which the balance between professional regulation, patient safety, and practitioner well-being is struck.

For some examples of well-being frameworks, see Boxes 1.10 and 1.11.

Box 1.10 Example 1: well-being framework—'Every Doctor, Every Setting' in Australia and New Zealand

In Australia, there has been recognition that the mental health and well-being of the medical profession is a national priority. Stakeholders regionally and nationally, with public and private providers, government regulatory agencies, universities, professional associations, and national mental health and suicide prevention agencies, have endorsed the 'Every Doctor, Every Setting' national framework to improve the well-being of the medical profession. The framework has brought together the best available evidence on what works to prevent and respond to mental ill-health and suicide as applied to the medical profession. It has been developed through a national working group, drawing on evidence review, consultation with professionals (including students), and other key stakeholders in healthcare. The framework prioritized five 'pillars' for intervention as shown in Fig. 1.6.

The systematized structure demonstrates how systems can improve the well-being of clinicians.

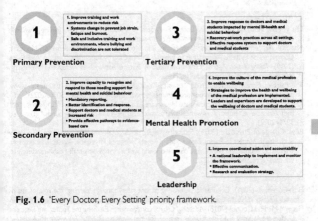

1 Primary Prevention
1. Improve training and work environments to reduce risk
• Systems change to prevent job strain, fatigue and burnout.
• Safe and inclusive training and work environments, where bullying and discrimination are not tolerated

3 Tertiary Prevention
3. Improve response to doctors and medical students impacted by mental ill-health and suicidal behaviour
• Recovery-at-work practices across all settings.
• Effective response system to support doctors and medical students

2 Secondary Prevention
2. Improve capacity to recognise and respond to those needing support for mental health and suicidal behaviour
• Mandatory reporting.
• Better identification and response.
• Support doctors and medical students at increased risk
• Provide effective pathways to evidence-based care

4 Mental Health Promotion
4. Improve the culture of the medical profession to enable wellbeing
• Strategies to improve the health and wellbeing of the medical profession are implemented.
• Leaders and supervisors are developed to support the wellbeing of doctors and medical students.

5 Leadership
5. Improve coordinated action and accountability
• A national leadership to implement and monitor the framework.
• Effective communication.
• Research and evaluation strategy.

Fig. 1.6 'Every Doctor, Every Setting' priority framework.

Box 1.11 Example 2: well-being framework—a systems approach to professional well-being in the US

In the US, a comprehensive review was undertaken to assess how to address clinical burnout and to facilitate well-being. The approach uses a Donabedian construct in which outcomes are determined by systemic and process factors. Systems include the external environment, the healthcare organization's culture, and the frontline care delivery environment which interact to impact the individual clinician. This impact will be mitigated or amplified by the processes in place and result in an outcome of either well-being or burnout (Fig. 1.7).

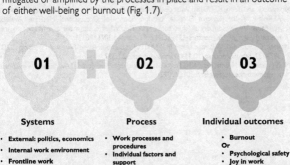

01 Systems
• External: politics, economics
• Internal work environment
• Frontline work

02 Process
• Work processes and procedures
• Individual factors and support

03 Individual outcomes
• Burnout
Or
• Psychological safety
• Joy in work
• Mental well-being

Fig. 1.7 A systems approach to well-being.

Interventions to facilitate well-being are required at each level, as well as acknowledging how factors may impact an individual in different ways.

Key interventions include a value-based system in which clinicians are valued and supported in a learning environment by compassionate leadership. Constant assessment of well-being and early intervention is important.

Signposting

Life in Mind Australia (n.d.). *Every Doctor, Every Setting: A National Framework*. [online] Available at: https://lifeinmind.org.au/every-doctor-every-setting (accessed 30/6/2022).

National Academies of Sciences, Engineering, and Medicine; National Academy of Medicine; Committee on Systems Approaches to Improve Patient Care by Supporting Clinician Well-Being (2019). *Taking Action Against Clinician Burnout: A Systems Approach to Professional Well-Being*. Washington, DC: National Academies Press.

The Point of Care Foundation (n.d.). *Schwartz Rounds Roles*. [online] Available at: https://www.pointofcarefoundation.org.uk/our-programmes/schwartz-rounds/ (accessed 30/6/2022).

The Schwartz Center for Compassionate Healthcare (n.d.). *Schwartz Rounds and Membership*. [online] Available at: https://www.theschwartzcenter.org/programs/schwartz-rounds/ (accessed 30/6/2022).

Royal College of Physicians (2015). *Setting Higher Standards. Work and Wellbeing in the NHS: Why Staff Health Matters to Patient Care*. London: Royal College of Physicians. Available at: https://www.rcplondon.ac.uk/guidelines-policy/work-and-wellbeing-nhs-why-staff-health-matters-pati ent-care (accessed 30/6/2022).

References

Firth-Cozens, J. (2001). Cultures for improving patient safety through learning: the role of teamwork. *Quality in Health Care: QHC*, 10(Suppl 2), ii26–ii31. https://doi.org/10.1136/qhc.0100026

General Medical Council (2018). *Adapting, Coping, Compromising: Exploring the Tactics and Decisions Doctors are Applying in a System Under Pressure*. [online] Available at: https://www.gmc-uk.org/-/media/documents/adapting-coping-compromising-quantitative-research-pt2-79705124.pdf (accessed 30/6/2022).

Gerada, C. (2018). Doctors, suicide and mental illness. *BJPsych Bulletin*, 42(4), 165–168. https://doi.org/10.1192/bjb.2018.11

Hall, L.H., Johnson, J., Watt, I., et al. (2016). Healthcare staff wellbeing, burnout, and patient safety: a systematic review. *PloS One*, 11(7), e0159015. https://doi.org/10.1371/journal.pone.0159015

Harvey, S.B., Epstein, R.M., Glozier, N., et al. (2021). Mental illness and suicide among physicians. *Lancet*, 398(10303), 920–930. https://doi.org/10.1016/S0140-6736(21)01596-8

Kay, M., Mitchell, G., Clavarino, A., et al. (2008). Doctors as patients: a systematic review of doctors' health access and the barriers they experience. *British Journal of General Practice*, 58(552), 501–508. https://doi.org/10.3399/bjgp08X319486

Kinman, G. and Teoh, K. (2018). *What Could Make a difference to the Mental Health of UK Doctors? A Review of the Research Evidence*. London: Society of Occupational Medicine. Available at: https://www.som.org.uk/sites/som.org.uk/files/What_could_make_a_difference_to_the_mental_health_of_UK_doctors_LTF_SOM.pdf (accessed 30/6/2022).

Maslach, C., Schaufeli, W.B., and Leiter, M.P. (2001). Job burnout. *Annual Review of Psychology*, 52(1), 397–422. https://doi.org/10.1146/annurev.psych.52.1.397

NHS Practitioner Health (n.d.). *NHS Practitioner Health Programme*. [online] Available at: www.practitionerhealth.nhs.uk (accessed 30/6/2022).

Organizational professionalism

What is organizational professionalism?

Doctors are familiar with the inherent required professionalism of the job, but healthcare organizations have an analogous code of behaviours and competencies which impact the patients and clinicians in the organization.

Why is this important?

The systems in which we practise influence our behaviour and organizational culture affects patients' outcomes. Good management of staff leads to higher-quality care, more satisfied patients, and lower patient mortality at lower cost. The more positive the experiences of staff in a healthcare organization, the better its outcomes. Staff level of engagement is especially crucial, being associated with patient satisfaction, mortality, infection rates, staff absence, and turnover. The role of the intersection of leadership, management, and education to positively influence the organizational culture of an institution, can therefore be key to the development of positive outcomes for patients and staff.

What is the theory?

Leadership has the profound ability to influence culture, as leaders have the power to control information and resources, reward or withdraw, and control the structure of the organization and its direction. The dissemination of these behaviours within the organization influences the perpetuation and ongoing leadership of the culture, be that positive or negative, which is the education piece. The management of individuals in the organization is perhaps the most powerful element of the leadership's ability to influence the culture.

How this works in practice

Leadership communicates and enacts an inspiring vision of the work they do, focused on high-quality compassionate care and using prominent language around a compelling vision, rather than a focus on targets, savings, and productivity.

Clear objectives aligned with this vision, in each directorate and department. Too many priorities mean blindness and paralysis. Objectives need to be challenging enough to be aspirational and thus motivating, and ideally measurable, to be able to give people feedback on their performance.

Good people management strongly influences how their patients experience their care. To influence patient care and experience, good staff management is key. Staff work pressure is associated with poor quality of care and poor staff well-being. Injury rates are associated with worse care. Implementation of good human resource management practices leads to a fall in mortality rates. The most important element of leadership on affecting an organization's culture is good staff management. We need fairness, transparency, and honesty.

Continually improving care at every level and including staff involvement, consultation, and learning from staff to find out the problems, identify solutions and innovations, set goals, and gather feedback.

Develop real teams that work effectively together across health and social care which are associated with fewer injuries, fewer errors, and less bullying. They require clear goals, roles, and communication across professional and organizational boundaries (see Inter-professionalism, p. 179).

Further reading

Egener, B., McDonald, W., Rosof, B., et al. (2012). Perspective: organizational professionalism: relevant competencies and behaviors. *Academic Medicine*, 87(5), 668–674. doi:10.1097/ACM.0b013e31824d4b67

West, M. (2013). *Developing Cultures of High-Quality Care*. [online] The Kings Fund. Available at: https://www.kingsfund.org.uk/audio-video/michael-west-developing-cultures-high-quality-care (accessed 30/6/2022).

West, M. (2014). *Changing Culture through Organisational Leadership*. [online] The Kings Fund. Available at: http://www.kingsfund.org.uk/publications/articles/changing-culture-through-collective-leadership-qa-michael-west (accessed 30/6/2022).

West, M., Dawson, J., Admasachew, L., et al. (2011). *NHS Staff Management and Health Service Quality*. London: Department of Health. Available at: https://assets.publishing.service.gov.uk/government/uploads/system/uploads/attachment_data/file/215455/dh_129656.pdf (accessed 30/6/2022).

Chapter 2

Management principles for clinical leaders

Introduction

Leadership is the ability to have a vision of how a department or team should develop and the ability to drive that change, in order to achieve desired results. Clinical leadership is when this role is taken by a clinician, bringing their unique world view.

Management is the activity of organizing the behaviour of a team towards desired objectives or results.

Over the past 20 years, hospital management has moved to include clinicians within the management structures, with the aim of bringing their perspective to the complex issues that need to be addressed. The emphasis is to put quality at the heart of health service provision, and for clinicians to develop a leadership and managerial role.

The NHS leadership framework provides a paradigm for the development of leadership skills (see Leadership frameworks, p. 16). There are also key skills which are focused on the practical day-to-day management within organizations, which are important to understand—and of which leaders will ideally have practical experience. This enables clinicians and managers to develop mutual respect and understanding for leadership, management, and clinical skills, as well as to position doctors as key drivers for change.

Appraisal and personal development plans

What are appraisal and personal development plans?

Appraisal is the process of facilitated self-review supported by information gathered from the full scope of an individual's work with the aim of maintaining and improving the quality of practice and key to demonstrating fitness to practise.

A personal development plan (PDP) is a key output of the appraisal process, expressing the individual's output and development needs for the coming year, with a clear plan to achieve these needs.

In the UK, the process of revalidation, introduced by the GMC, relies heavily on annual appraisal to inform a 5-yearly review of fitness to practise. Evidence of compliance with the GMC's *Good Medical Practice* guidance has to be provided within the NHS, private practice, and any other settings where a doctor practises.

What is the theory?

Appraisal is an annual structured process to review overall practice, an opportunity for reflection, to assess needs for development, and to inform the ongoing quality and safety of a clinician's work or similar. The idea is that this starts at an individual level and assures the quality of clinical staff organizationally and from the perspective of the profession (regulatory). Appraisal relies on a number of processes (e.g. reflection, feedback on performance, developing insight) that are commonly used when regulators and professional bodies in other jurisdictions assess the fitness to practise of doctors (Brennan et al., 2017).

The GMC in the UK identifies four domains for review and reflection:
1. Knowledge, skills, and performance.
2. Safety and quality.
3. Communication, partnership, and teamwork.
4. Maintaining trust.

The PDP represents the main output from the appraisal which lists the developmental needs for the following year. Dates for achievements and expected outcomes are set, and once completed, the appraisal can be signed off by the appraiser and appraisee.

Why is this important?

Appraisal is important as it facilitates self-reflection on performance and self-identification of developmental needs. This can enhance the quality of professional work by ensuring the planning of professional development. The appraisal meeting enables doctors to discuss their practice and performance in order to meet the principles and values set out in *Good Medical Practice*. The key outcome is ensuring doctors are working productively in line with the priorities of their organizations.

Appraisal informs professional regulation and revalidation where required.

Components of the appraisal process

An appraisal is a frank and open discussion by the appraiser and the appraisee (Box 2.1). Both appraiser and appraisee need to respect time, be prepared, and to be able to look for strengths as well as areas for potential development. The appraiser and appraisee will together look at the evidence and jointly decide on any development requirements and actions to be taken.

Box 2.1 Appraisal process

1. Inputs to appraisal:
   a. Personal information.
   b. Scope and nature of work: to include all clinical, managerial, educational, research, voluntary, and academic roles.
   c. Supporting information: 360-degree review, continuing professional development requirements of Royal College, quality improvement activity, significant events, feedback from colleagues, feedback from patients, review of complaints and compliments, and proof of mandatory training.
   d. Review of previous year's PDP and development activities.
   e. Achievements, challenges, and aspirations.
2. Confidential appraisal discussion.
3. Outputs of appraisal:
   a. PDP.
   b. Summary of appraisal.
   c. Appraiser's statement.
4. Post-appraisal sign off by doctor and appraiser.

Appraisee

See Box 2.2.

Box 2.2 Actions for appraisee

Reflect

- Appraisal encourages constant reflective practice and preparation should be an ongoing process.
- Maintain a reflective diary and record of learning.
- Maintain and collect supportive evidence throughout the year.
- Allow time to prepare for the appraisal process.
- Reflect on the appraisal year.
- Gather examples of your achievements and behaviours in line with the Trust values.
- Understand the correct paperwork or electronic record required for your role.

Prepare

- Discuss your appraisal in advance with your line manager.
- Obtain feedback from colleagues and stakeholders on what you have achieved in the past appraisal year and how you have done it.
- Gather evidence of training you have completed.
- Undergo a 360-degree review if required.
- Gather patient feedback.
- Ensure you have an up-to-date CPD record.
- Check your professional registration.
- Obtain up-to-date forms from the organization regarding any complaints or disciplinary actions, as well as 'Transfer of Information' forms from independent hospitals where you do not regularly work.

In the UK, trainee doctors are appraised through the Annual Review of Competence Progression (ARCP) mechanism.

Appraiser

Medical appraisers should have completed a recognized medical appraisal training course.

Appraisal documentation and outcomes should be kept for at least 5 years (and potentially for the duration of a career). The outcomes of an appraisal can be used to provide weight to job planning processes and professional development requests. See Box 2.3.

Box 2.3 Actions by appraiser

- Read the documentation ahead of time.
- Look for strengths on which the appraisee can build.
- Consider areas for development in a positive way.
- Be always respectful of the appraisee.
- Allow a two-way discussion.
- Listen and reflect.
- Facilitate self-reflection by the appraisee.
- Allow the appraisee to lead on the PDP.
- Be realistic.
- Always keep to time.

Signposting

Academy of Medical Royal Colleges (2014). *Appraisal for Revalidation: A Guide to the Process*. [online] Available at: https://www.aomrc.org.uk/wp-content/uploads/2016/04/Appraisal_Revalidation _Guide_Process_0714.pdf (accessed 3/10/2021).

General Medical Council (2019). *Good Medical Practice*. London: General Medical Council. Available at: www.gmc-uk.org/guidance/good_medical_practice.asp (accessed 3/10/2021).

General Medical Council (2020). *Supporting Information for Appraisal and Revalidation*. [online] Available at: https://www.gmc-uk.org/-/media/documents/RT___Supporting_information_ for_appraisal_and_revalidation___DC5485.pdf_55024594.pdf (accessed 3/10/2021).

Further reading

Brennan, N., Bryce, M., Pearson, M., et al. (2017). Towards an understanding of how appraisal of doctors produces its effects: a realist review. *Medical Education*, 51(10), 1002–1013. doi:10.1111/ medu.13348

Job planning

What is job planning?

Job planning is an annual prospective agreement between a doctor and their employer. It sets out duties, responsibilities, and objectives. Its overall purpose is to review the range of work activities undertaken and to ensure that the workload is appropriately planned and remunerated (Box 2.4).

Job planning should be aligned with national, professional, and the employer's local needs and guidance, and therefore requires a partnership approach between the doctor and their employer. It provides an opportunity for the clinician and the manager to agree clinical goals as well as to come to an agreement on how to continually improve quality and safety of care.

The aim is to ensure that the work can be undertaken in a manner that protects both the patient and the clinician, while building on safety of care as a key focus.

Box 2.4 Principles of job planning

Job planning should take the following principles into account:
- Professionalism of being a doctor.
- Outcome focused for benefit of patients.
- Synchronized with system-wide objectives.
- Consistent with team values.
- Transparent, fair, and just.
- Flexible and adaptable to changing needs.
- Agreed as a compact and not imposed to deliver the personal goals of the individual and the system as a whole.
- Enables a good work–life balance.
- Enhances psychological safety.

Why is this important?

Job planning is part of the appraisal and revalidation process. It documents the realistic workload and helps to prioritize work that needs to be done. It helps doctors support the wider objectives of the service and meet the

Box 2.5 Components of a job plan

The job plan detail includes:
- a timetable of activities (Table 2.1)
- a summary of the total number of programmed activities (PAs) of each type in the timetable; a PA is usually 4 hours in duration
- on-call arrangements (i.e. supplement category and rota)
- a list of agreed SMART (Specific, Measurable, Achievable, Realistic, and Time-focused) objectives
- a list of supporting resources necessary to achieve objectives
- a description of additional responsibilities to the wider NHS and profession (including external duties)
- arrangements for additional PAs
- details of regular private work
- accountability arrangements
- signing off and review.

needs of patients and the provision of safe and high-quality care. If effective, job planning can improve service delivery. From the individual's perspective, job planning ensures that the requirements of the post are within working time regulations and makes best use of the clinician's skills as well as protecting development time.

Personal objectives

A good job plan incorporates job content, time and service commitments, as well as personal objectives. It ties in with PDPs that form part of the appraisal process (see Appraisal and personal development plans, p. 37).

Clear objectives provide focus for doctors and managers and help with both service provision and quality improvements. Objectives should be SMART.

Signposting

NHS Employers (2017). *A Guide to Consultant Job Planning*. London: BMA and NHS. Available at: https://www.nhsemployers.org/pay-pensions-and-reward/medical-staff/consultants-and-dental-consultants/job-planning (accessed 3/10/2021).

NHS England (2020). *E-job Planning*. [online] Available at: https://www.england.nhs.uk/wp-content/uploads/2020/09/e-job-planning-guidance.pdf (accessed 3/10/2021).

Table 2.1 Example of a radiologist's detailed job plan

Day	Time	Site	Work	Category	PAs	Hours
Mon	09:00–13:00	Hospital 1	Screen reading	Direct clinical contact (DCC)	1.000	4.0
	13:00–17:00	Hospital 1	Symptomatic breast clinic	DCC	1.000	4.0
	17:00–18:00	Hospital 1	Multidisciplinary team (MDT) preparation	DCC	0.250	1.0
Tues	07:30–10:00	Hospital 1	MDT meeting	DCC	0.625	2.5
	10:00–12:00	Hospital 1	Supporting professional activities (SPA)	SPA	0.500	2.0
	12:00–14:30	Hospital 1	Computed tomography (CT), magnetic resonance imaging (MRI) reporting	DCC	0.625	2.5
Wed	09:00–13:30	Hospital 1	Assessment clinic	DCC	1.125	4.5
	13:30–14:00	Travel	Cross-site travel	DCC	0.125	0.5
	14:00–17:00	Hospital 2	Inpatient ultrasound	DCC	0.750	3.0
	17:00–20:30	Hospital 2	Inpatient CT/ultrasound Alternate weeks	DCC	0.500	2.0
Thurs	09:00–13:00	Hospital 1	Symptomatic breast clinic	DCC	1.000	4.0
	13:00–17:00	Hospital 1	Follow-up ultrasound clinic	DCC	1.000	4.0
	17:00–18:00	Hospital 1	MRI reporting	DCC	0.250	1.0
			Clinic cross-cover	DCC	0.250	1.0
			Off-site SPA	SPA	1.000	4.0
			On-call (1 in 15)	DCC	1.000	4.0
			Intensity supplement on-call 3%			
					11.000	44.0

Performance management

What is performance management?

Performance management is a term used to describe improving the effectiveness of services, teams, and individuals. Here we focus primarily on the environment for performance management and how it relates to the individual. Chapter 4 describes system performance and values-based health systems as an approach at the level of a service and organization (see Measuring system performance, p. 103, and Creating a value-based healthcare system, p. 109).

Performance management of individuals is a process by which managers and employees work together to plan, monitor, and review an employee's work objectives and overall contribution to the organization. It is a continuous process designed to ensure that the performance of an individual employee contributes to the goals of the individual teams and organization (Fig. 2.1). Doctors might be involved in performance managing others or may be performance managed themselves.

Why is this important?

Good performance management helps everyone in an organization to know what the organization is trying to achieve and the employee's role in helping the organization achieve its goals. It defines the skill competencies and standards of performance that an employee needs to fulfil their role.

Performance management can assist the employee to perform well as an individual and contribute to the development of the organization. It also can identify when performance problems arise and determine what can be done to improve performance.

What is the theory?

Locke and Latham's (2002) proposed goal-setting forms the basis for performance management. It is based on the premise that conscious goals affect action where goals are considered the object or aim of an action. The theory was developed in the corporate world and proposes that well-defined objectives, such as 'increase sales by 20%', are more effective than less well-defined objectives, such as 'complete your work to a higher standard'. They also emphasized that the best way to feel motivated is to set goals that individuals are not sure they could 100% achieve—as opposed to being unachievable. The sense of accomplishment associated with achieving is reinforcing and developmental in terms of performance. Performance management is a 'carrot' process rather than a 'stick'.

In individual performance management, application of this theory to set realistically achievable targets through a formal process of review is the overall aim.

Characteristics of a successful performance management system

A successful system will communicate the organization or departmental vision to all employees and set targets for departmental, team, and individual performance in keeping with wide corporate objectives. The system conducts regular formal reviews of progress to identify, develop, and reward outcomes and evaluate the performance management process to improve effectiveness.

Setting outcome goals

Clearly define the results that would satisfy completing the goal. Link the goal to the wider organizational (or departmental) goal and ensure the goal is achievable but also difficult enough to motivate performance. Finally, limit to several goals only.

How does this work in practice?

There are three aspects to planning an individual's performance:
- Identifying objectives which the employee is expected to achieve.
- Highlighting competencies or behaviours—the way in which employees work towards their objectives.
- Charting personal development—the development employees need in order to achieve objectives and realize their potential.

In practice, this is a two-way process, and regular dialogue between line managers and their team members is at the heart of performance management. Managers should discuss work as it goes along by holding regular informal meetings about:
- how the employee is doing in terms of objectives and competencies and whether anything could be added to the employee's record of achievement
- identifying competencies that could be further enhanced
- areas to work on and any concerns about performance—these can feed into the employee's development plan.

Reviewing performance typically has three elements:
- Regular informal meetings, where line managers discuss current work and development. Close links with human resources are generally kept with good note-keeping and adhering to the local policies.
- Formal interim meetings to discuss progress against performance plans.
- Annual appraisal reviews, where the work of the year is discussed and feedback given.

For some tips for success, see Box 2.6.

Box 2.6 Tips for success

Promoting a workplace that encourages feedback and encourages staff to develop the improvement and development process facilitates the improvement of a service.

Senior clinicians need to consider their role in the performance management process, including staff to whom they do not have direct authoritative management responsibility, and how they might be able to provide the positive feedback outcomes (or even rewards) to motivate teams further.

Tips for giving feedback:
- Try to give feedback as close to the witnessed event as possible, in private if appropriate.
- Ask the view of the individual to whom you are giving feedback.
- Give specific feedback about effective and ineffective behaviours.
- Avoid focusing on personal characteristics—concentrate on what they did or did not do (utilize examples).
- Spend time working with the individual to plan to address any needs that have arisen from the feedback.
- Offer help in achieving development needs and provide resources where appropriate.

How do you do this already?

Effective implementation of appraisal and work-based assessment promotes the development of the individual and this contributes to the performance of the team, department, and organization.

Understanding performance difficulties in doctors

An individual's performance is affected by a complex interplay of both personal and situational factors including, but not limited to, organizational culture, physical environment, teamwork, personal life, and leadership. Workload, sleep, health, and shift patterns can all have an impact on clinical performance. Well-being and psychological safety are an essential part of ensuring there is good performance.

The majority of doctors work hard, strive to achieve high standards, and provide excellent services for their patients. In some circumstances, doctors may find themselves unable to perform their duties and it is inevitable that some fail to meet the required and expected standards.

Every doctor has a duty to report any concerns they might have about their own, or a colleague's, performance. If required, this needs to be escalated to the appropriate line manager of the department.

Training budgets are usually available, should specific learning needs be identified. These needs should be included in the PDP.

If there are concerns about a doctor's performance, there are various considerations to take into account, such as physical and mental health, education and training, leadership, workload, and teamworking abilities.

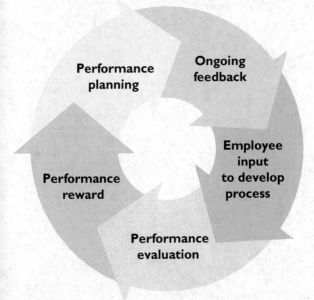

Fig. 2.1 Performance management cycle.

Further reading

Locke, E.A. and Latham, G.P. (2002). Building a practically useful theory of goal setting and task motivation: a 35-year odyssey. *American Psychologist*, 57(9), 705–717. https://doi.org/10.1037/0003-066X.57.9.705

NHS Employers (2021). *People Performance Management Toolkit*. [online] Available at: https://www.nhsemployers.org/sites/default/files/2021-07/People-Performance-Management-Toolkit.pdf (accessed 3/10/2021).

Powell, A. and Davies, H. (2016). *Managing Doctors, Doctors Managing*. [online] Nuffield Trust. Available at: https://www.nuffieldtrust.org.uk/files/2017-01/doctors-managers-web-final.pdf (accessed 3/10/2021).

Trebble, T.M., Heyworth, N., Clarke, N. et al. (2014). Managing hospital doctors and their practice: what can we learn about human resource management from non-healthcare organizations? *BMC Health Services Research*, 14, 566. DOI: 10.1186/s12913-014-0566-5

Time management

What is time management?

Time management describes techniques and habits that enable you to make the best use of the valuable resource that is your time. It is not how to pack more activity into your day; it is how to spend your time on the right things at the right time.

Why is time management important?

A clinician's time is an expensive, limited, and valuable resource. Senior clinicians are usually given a degree of autonomy over how they use their time as they are expected to manage their working day and make the best use of available resources within continually changing systems. In so doing, they must demonstrate flexibility, decisiveness, and a high level of organization.

The job planning process allocates the time that is available and the good use of that time is important to achieve both individual and organizational objectives.

How does this work in practice?

Prioritization

By considering the urgency and importance of a new task, one can place it into one of four quadrants in the time management matrix (Fig. 2.2). This allows one to sequence tasks into order of priority. One then transfers to a diary and commit to action them. The matrix allows one to prioritize activities in a logical manner so that time can be allocated.

Important tasks have an outcome which helps us to achieve our goals (e.g. high-quality patient care, PDP).

Urgent tasks demand immediate attention.

- Quadrant 1 tasks are classed *urgent and important* and require immediate action.

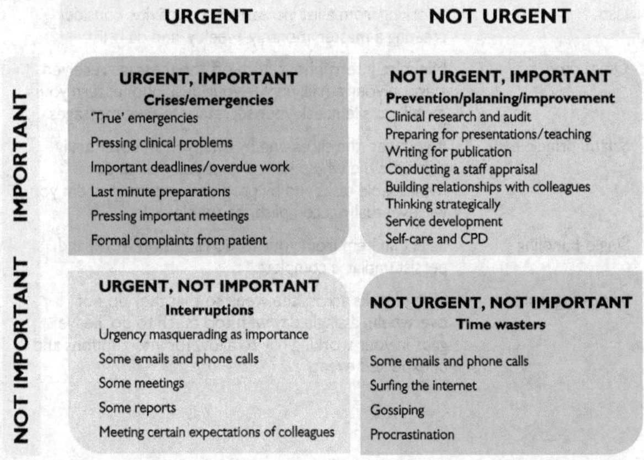

	URGENT	**NOT URGENT**
IMPORTANT	**URGENT, IMPORTANT** **Crises/emergencies** 'True' emergencies Pressing clinical problems Important deadlines/overdue work Last minute preparations Pressing important meetings Formal complaints from patient	**NOT URGENT, IMPORTANT** **Prevention/planning/improvement** Clinical research and audit Preparing for presentations/teaching Writing for publication Conducting a staff appraisal Building relationships with colleagues Thinking strategically Service development Self-care and CPD
NOT IMPORTANT	**URGENT, NOT IMPORTANT** **Interruptions** Urgency masquerading as importance Some emails and phone calls Some meetings Some reports Meeting certain expectations of colleagues	**NOT URGENT, NOT IMPORTANT** **Time wasters** Some emails and phone calls Surfing the internet Gossiping Procrastination

Fig. 2.2 A time management matrix.

- Quadrant 2 tasks are *not urgent but are important* and should be completed every day. These are critical for a clear vision, balanced life, discipline, control, and fewer and fewer crises.
- Quadrant 3 activities are *urgent but are not important* and they should be restricted.
- Quadrant 4 tasks are those which are *not urgent and not important* and should not be undertaken.

Additional time-management techniques are available and can be chosen to suit preference and situation. A summary of these is available in Table 2.2. For some tips for success, see Box 2.7.

Table 2.2 Additional time management techniques

Technique	Action to take
Avoid procrastination	If you have a tendency to procrastinate about certain tasks, make a point of doing them first to get them out of the way
Batching	Dedicate blocks of time to similar tasks (e.g. emails, phone calls, dictations), in order to decrease distraction and increase productivity
Decision-making	Make decisions quickly, as problems arise, or identify a time for the decision to be made and set a reminder
Diaries	It is important to choose a type of diary that works best for you—electronic, paper, etc. Diaries must not be a barrier but an enabler
Energy peaks	Work on your most important/difficult tasks at your energy peaks (the times of day when you are most alert and productive), e.g. writing a report in the evening may take you 2 hours compared to 1 hour if you were to wake up early
Lists	Working from a list increases productivity; consider creating a master, monthly, weekly, and daily list
Quiet time	Minimize interruptions; turn off the message received alert on your email; unplug your desk phone; turn your mobile to silent; ask your secretary to take messages
Salami principle	If you 'eat' the slices one by one, you will eventually consume the whole 'salami'. Set yourself small manageable tasks and by progressing through them you will eventually accomplish the whole task
Single-handling	Select an item from your to-do list, begin work, and persist until it is complete
Spreading tasks	Spread tasks across the week so that they do not overwhelm a single day with too much to do. Leave gaps in your working day to allow for interruptions and unexpected events

Table 2.2   (Contd.)

Technique	Action to take
Time log	Complete a job planning and ask yourself:
	• What activities do I not need to do?
	• What am I doing that someone else can do?
	• What can I do more efficiently?
	• What do I do that wastes others' time?
Transition time	Time spent commuting or waiting is an invaluable resource for answering emails (if technology allows), reading, planning, and reflecting
Two-minute rule	Complete tasks that take 2 minutes or less immediately; this will give you momentum and free up your mind to focus on other activities
Workspace	An organized and clean workspace can increase productivity. Invest time in setting up your workspace(s)

Box 2.7 Tips for success

- Time management skills can only develop in parallel with other management skills, such as delegation.
- Some techniques/habits will be more helpful than others and none will provide the full solution. Every person is different and his or her time management problems will be unique.
- Once you have identified your own preferred way of working, it is important to persevere with it, to embed it in your daily routine. Challenge negative thinking. You will never know whether a technique is effective until you try it.

Further reading

Christie, S. (2012). *Effective Time Management Skills for Doctors.* London: BPP Learning Media Ltd.

Covey, S. (2004). *The 7 Habits of Highly Effective People.* London: Simon and Schuster UK Ltd.

Pitre, C., Pettit, K., Ladd, L., et al. (2018). Physician time management. *MedEdPORTAL*, 14, 10681–10687. https://doi.org/10.15766/mep_2374-8265.10681

Rimmer, A. (2019). How do I improve my time management skills? *BMJ*, 366, l5322. doi:10.1136/bmj.l5322

Chairing meetings

What is the role of the chair?

A chair ensures that a meeting runs efficiently and that all relevant matters are discussed. It is essential that everyone's views are heard, clear decisions are made, and that the meeting runs to time.

Why is this important?

Meetings are essential for clinical and managerial practice and can be:

* a regular, day-to-day activity (for responding to queries that need a rapid response, managing daily concerns, or maintaining channels of communication)
* less frequent, in-depth gatherings (for responding to the demand for change and generating new ways of working).

How does this work in practice?

A successful meeting requires planning and has three phases.

Before the meeting

* Involve key personnel at an early stage of planning.
* Ensure the purpose of the meeting (e.g. information sharing, consultation, decision-making) is known to attendees in advance.
* Allocate sufficient resources to the meeting (e.g. time, venue, suitable layout, audiovisual aids).
* Prepare a clear and inclusive agenda that can be effectively addressed in the time available; prioritize important items.
* Circulate the agenda, supporting papers (e.g. minutes from a previous meeting), and, if necessary, a venue map in advance.
* Read/discuss the background information and consider potential conflicts of interest (e.g. competing priorities).
* Have a contingency for non-attendance of members.
* Arrange seating to maximize interaction and contribution.

During the meeting

* Start and end on time.
* Ensure that good notes are taken and, if needed, appoint an individual to take minutes or notes.
* Agree the ground rules. These include refraining from interrupting and making personal remarks, and limiting arguments to the issues being discussed. The chair will highlight when a discussion has drifted off topic.
* Gain commitment to the agenda: 'We must achieve x and y.'
* Read the minutes or notes and action points of the last meeting or invite members to do so; are there any additions or corrections?
* Allow sufficient time for each agenda item.
* Review progress on action points from any previous meetings.
* Seek full and active participation of everyone in the meeting and ensure that all views are heard, valued, and summarized.
* Invite and discuss alternative viewpoints and outcomes to avoid focusing down on a solution too quickly.
* Consider the advantages, disadvantages, and impact of proposed changes.
* Steer discussions in a structured fashion and keep them realistic.

After the meeting
- Summarize key points and decisions and draw up an explicit timed action plan to identify who will do what, by when.
- Agree the agenda, time, and location for the next meeting.
- Thank all participants for their contribution.
- Circulate the minutes to all members within an agreed time and no more than 2 weeks after the meeting.

Handling individual agenda items
It can be helpful to think of each item as a diamond shape as shown in Fig. 2.3.

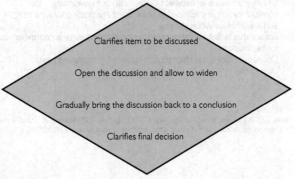

Fig. 2.3 Handling individual agenda items.

The chair of the meeting:
- clarifies the issues to be discussed (the top of the diamond)
- opens up the discussion and encourages it to widen (the body of the diamond)
- gradually brings the discussion back to a conclusion
- clarifies the final decision (the bottom of the diamond).

Virtual meetings

The COVID-19 pandemic has brought new challenges in chairing a meeting, with the default position often being that meetings occur online using a variety of different interfaces.

The Kings Fund has produced guidance for attendees and chairs of meetings to ensure that they run smoothly and consider as much as possible the difference in interaction that this interface produces. The key is to keep presentations short as attention span is 5–10 minutes, promote discussion by using breakout rooms for small group discussion, and be inclusive by ensuing all have a way to participate be it vocally or in the chat facility. Active listening is important as this integrates facts, feelings, and intention of the participants.

For some tips for success, see Box 2.8.

Box 2.8 Tips for success

You can encourage participation by the following:

- Asking open and searching questions.
- Using active listening such as nodding, eye contact, smiling, reflecting, summarizing, paraphrasing.
- Gently inviting others to elaborate, for example, 'Perhaps you could explain …', or offer alternative views.
- Being alert to and acknowledging those who wish to be brought into the debate.
- Chairing provides an excellent opportunity for developing communication and leadership skills; invite feedback on your strengths and weaknesses when chairing.
- Ensure that task-orientated meetings have appropriate authority to make decisions.
- Do not use being the chair to dominate the meeting with your own ideas.

Signposting

Hulks, S. (2020). *Leading Virtual Meetings*. [online] The Kings Fund. 2020 Available at: https://www.kingsfund.org.uk/publications/leading-virtual-meetings-top-tips (accessed 3/10/2021).

Giving feedback

What is feedback?

A two-way process in which a line manager, educational supervisor, or group appropriately share with the line manager or learner information based on observation, with the aim of reaching a defined goal and improving performance.

Why is feedback important?

Positive feedback boosts morale and reinforces preferred ways of working. Feedback about unhelpful behaviour allows the recipient to improve their practice or target their learning. Feedback is a crucial component of educational supervision, for example, workplace-based assessments and leadership and management development, especially if integrated into the appraisal/job planning/personal development cycle. In the UK, patient and colleague multi-source feedback should be undertaken by doctors registered with the GMC at least once in each 5-year revalidation cycle.

What is the theory?

Feedback is a developmental process which allows individuals to measure how well their performance is matching expectations. External feedback was recognized by philosophers such as Aristotle as being vital in an individual learning when they are doing something well as opposed to poorly. Educational theorists have identified ways in which feedback should occur, at which times, for maximum benefit and efficacy.

How does this work in practice?

Feedback can be informal (e.g. on the job) or formal (e.g. end of attachment interviews). Effective feedback is:

* **B**alanced (highlights helpful aspects of performance and behaviour as well as areas that need improvement)
* **O**bserved (limited to observable decisions and actions and not based on inferences about motives)
* **O**bjective (delivered in descriptive, non-evaluative and non-judgemental language)
* **S**pecific (based on specific behaviours rather than general performance)
* **T**imely (planned, expected, and given as close to the event as possible to ensure accuracy and effectiveness).

Receiving feedback

Individual responses to feedback vary and may be negative (e.g. anger, denial, blame, rationalization).

* When receiving feedback, allow yourself to experience an emotional response.
* When you are ready, consider which aspects of the feedback might actually be true—avoid the urge to act on any negative thoughts or feelings.
* What might you do to make the changes asked for or implied?

Fig. 2.4 outlines the ways in which competence and feedback can be related. For some tips for success, see Box 2.9.

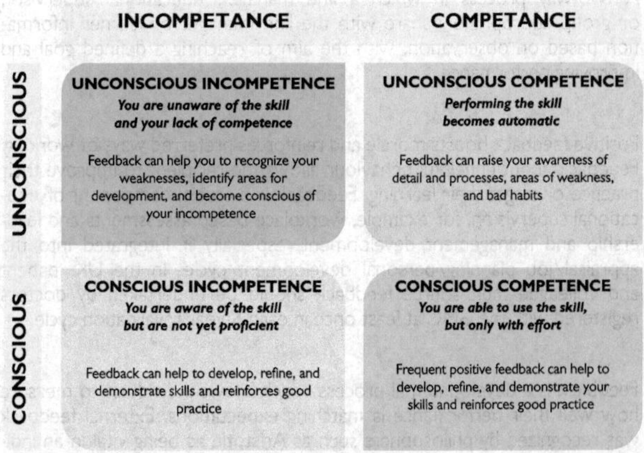

	INCOMPETANCE	COMPETANCE
UNCONSCIOUS	**UNCONSCIOUS INCOMPETENCE** *You are unaware of the skill and your lack of competence* Feedback can help you to recognize your weaknesses, identify areas for development, and become conscious of your incompetence	**UNCONSCIOUS COMPETENCE** *Performing the skill becomes automatic* Feedback can raise your awareness of detail and processes, areas of weakness, and bad habits
CONSCIOUS	**CONSCIOUS INCOMPETENCE** *You are aware of the skill but are not yet proficient* Feedback can help to develop, refine, and demonstrate skills and reinforces good practice	**CONSCIOUS COMPETENCE** *You are able to use the skill, but only with effort* Frequent positive feedback can help to develop, refine, and demonstrate your skills and reinforces good practice

Fig. 2.4 Feedback and competence.

Box 2.9 Tips for success

- The broader the range of people giving feedback, the more rounded and useful it becomes.
- Providing false feedback to spare someone's feelings is pointless and ultimately detrimental, as unhelpful behaviour will not be highlighted or changed.
- Feedback is essential to help us progress from unconscious incompetence to unconscious competence (Fig. 2.4).

Further reading

Cantillon, P. and Sargeant, J. (2008). Giving feedback in clinical settings. *BMJ*, 337, a1961. DOI:10.1136/bmj.a1961

King J. (1999). Giving feedback. *BMJ*, 318, S2-7200. https://doi.org/10.1136/bmj.318.7200.2

Negotiation

What is negotiation?

Negotiation is conferring with others in order to reach agreement through compromise.

Why is this important?

Negotiation skills are helpful in many situations:

- Multidisciplinary team working (e.g. improving relationships and collaboration).
- Quality improvement (e.g. implementing a new care pathway requires influencing skills and identifying and overcoming areas of resistance).
- Team and organizational leadership and management.
- Job planning (e.g. negotiating a change in practice).

What is the theory?

Negotiation involves 'giving' something in exchange for 'getting' something you want. There is a theory of negotiation which suggests a focus on interests and cooperation wherever possible, revealing information to create maximum value, while at the same time attempting to calculate the risks and rewards of sharing that information with the counterpart.

How does this work in practice?

Preparation

- Know the facts.
- If you are representing a group, understand their attitudes and opinions.
- Anticipate the other side's likely priorities and arguments.
- Identify the range of outcomes with which you would be happy—ask:
    - 'What do I want to achieve?' and 'Why do I want to achieve that?' (i.e. to reveal your bigger picture goals).
    - 'What is my ideal outcome?' (i.e. those who enter negotiations with higher aspirations attain better outcomes).
    - 'What is my 'stretch target?' (i.e. a justifiable outcome with which you would be very happy).
    - 'What is my minimum acceptable outcome?' (i.e. that is still worthwhile to you with reference to your bigger picture goals).
- Identify potentially negotiable points:
    - 'What are the different variables?'
    - 'What are my preferred outcomes for each?'
    - 'What do I have that the other party wants and is easy for me to give away?'

Clarification at the start

- Clarify the other party's position.
- State your ideal outcome and potential negotiable points.
- Listen for and name mixed messages.
- Reflect, summarize, and clarify where necessary.

Exchange of opinion and persuasion

- Delineate crucial points for both parties.
- Advance the discussion.
- Limit interruptions.
- Challenge where appropriate.

Encourage movement
- Keep your outcomes in mind.
- Be creative—negotiation is a problem-solving exercise:
  - Lay both parties' agendas, resources, and constraints on the table.
  - Try to find a solution that achieves both parties' agendas, given both parties' constraints and resources.
- Concede in small steps from your ideal outcome.
- Adjourn, if necessary, as both parties can then discuss and modify their position.

Completing the deal
- Summarize, verbally and in writing, what has been achieved and what is left to complete.

For some tips for success, see Box 2.10.

Box 2.10 Tips for success

Communication skills
- Ask questions to reveal information or 'unknown unknowns'.
- Listen deeply to understand the leverage points and how best to convey your message.
- Be clear and effective when articulating your message.

Emotional intelligence
Emotional intelligence is the ability to recognize and respond to your emotions and those of others, when in a negotiation this will allow you to:
- be confident and at your peak performance
- remain dispassionate, calm, and logical
- manage the other party's emotions
- inspire the other party with the deal you are offering.

Further reading

Souza, B.D. and Barton, A. (2014). The art of negotiating as a doctor. *BMJ*, 349, g6662. https://doi.org/10.1136/bmj.g6662

Walsh, K. (2015). Negotiation skills for medical educators. *Journal of Graduate Medical Education*, 7(1), 12–13. https://doi:10.4300/JGME-D-14-00328.1

Delegation

What is delegation?

Delegation is a means of sharing out or transferring responsibilities to others.

Why is it important?

Delegation can benefit the delegator, the person delegated to, and the team as a whole. When undertaken properly, delegation can free up the time of the delegator to focus on more important tasks that cannot be delegated. It can stretch and develop members of the team.

When colleagues are trusted with greater responsibility, they apply extra 'discretionary effort' to fulfil the task and develop their personal skills, expertise, and confidence in their abilities to the benefit of all. Finally, this can increase their commitment to the issue, foster good working relationships, and improve morale.

What is the theory?

No leader or manager could or should undertake all the activities expected of him or her; it is inevitable that some matters will need to be delegated. Ultimately, responsibility rests with the delegator but the person to whom the task is delegated is responsible to the delegator for carrying this out.

How does it work in practice?

- Identify the right thing to delegate (see Time management and prioritization, p. 47).
- *Set outcomes:* be clear about what needs to be done.
- *Identify an individual to whom to delegate:* they must possess, or need to develop, suitable skills, experience, and motivation to complete the task.
- *Hold a briefing meeting:*
  - Explain the task and clarify the desired outcome.
  - Describe the context, including the reasons for delegation and the importance of the task at large.
  - Agree the resources needed to carry out the work (e.g. finance, training, equipment, cooperation of others).
  - Confirm that instructions have been understood.
  - If required for the task, make others aware that you have delegated your authority.
- *Monitoring:* be available throughout the task to give support, advice, and guidance.
- *Review:* at the end of the task, evaluate the results.

There is valuable literature regarding delegation of clinical work within the nursing profession (see 'Further reading'), much of which is also applicable to doctors. The principles of delegation of non-clinical tasks and clinical tasks remain the same, although regulatory frameworks and skillsets must be borne in mind, and advice/guidance should be sought from the relevant professional regulator.

For some tips for success, see Box 2.11.

Box 2.11 Tips for success

- Not all tasks are suitable for delegation (e.g. serious conflict management).
- Appropriate allocation of tasks requires awareness of your team's knowledge and skills.
- Inappropriate allocation may result in failure of task completion and:
  - a need for the task to be reassigned
  - reduced confidence in, and of, the individual
  - feelings of resentment towards the delegator.
- Reflect on your relationship to delegation—are your beliefs and assumptions holding you back? Common unhelpful beliefs include:
  - 'I cannot trust anyone to do the job properly'
  - 'It takes too long to explain—it is quicker to do it myself'
  - 'I don't want to burden my team with extra responsibilities.'

Further reading

Royal College of Nursing (2017). *Accountability and Delegation*. London: Royal College of Nursing. Available at: https://www.rcn.org.uk/professional-development/accountability-and-delegation (accessed 3/10/2021).

General Medical Council (2019). *Good Medical Practice: Delegation and Referral*. London: General Medical Council. Available at: https://www.gmc-uk.org/ethical-guidance/ethical-guidance-for-doctors/delegation-and-referral (accessed 3/10/2021).

Business planning

What is business planning?

Business planning is the process of setting out the strategic direction of a proposed or existing project, team, or organization. It takes into account the financial, organizational, and political aspects of any development. Examples could be a reorganization of an existing clinical service or the way it is delivered, or the creation of a department.

Why is it important?

Doctors, nurses, and other healthcare practitioners are often well placed to identify opportunities for service improvement. Any significant service redesign or development of a new service will have financial, organizational, and political implications. The ability to make an effective business plan is a critical skill for clinical leaders who wish to implement their ideas.

What is the theory?

A business plan provides a guide for managing the start-up and operations of a service, comprising a formal statement of the objectives of the proposed change, the reasons why they are believed attainable, and the plan for reaching those goals. At a minimum, it includes a description of the activity and a comprehensive breakdown of costs, benefits (both financial and in activity and quality), and revenues to the organization.

   The process of preparing the plan can help to clarify financial and operational detail and should provide convincing justification to stakeholders of the merit, both in service, clinical, and financial terms, of the proposed change. It will be used as a decision-making tool as to whether to support the project (financially or otherwise) by the leaders of the organization and their senior financial officers, whose backing will be critical to the success of the project.

Key components of a business plan

Many healthcare organizations will have their own internal templates for the preparation of business plans. Below is a fairly standard structure to a business plan but this is not fixed and may be adapted to the requirements of the project (see also Box 2.12). Components typically included are:

Box 2.12 Characteristics of a successful business plan

- Clarity of writing.
- Objectivity.
- Clearly definable benefit—for example, lowered costs or novel utility for reasonable expenditure.
- Consistency/coherence—reads as if 'from one voice'.
- Accuracy—be clear about any assumptions.
- Key people—should be named where possible, with evidence that they are appropriately skilled for their role.

Executive summary

A good business plan starts with a summary of the proposed project. This should be a statement outlining the purpose and goals and to show how these goals will be realized, including a detailed marketing or communication strategy. Emphasis should be on benefits of the proposed change to the service/patients, relevant investment requirements, and potential resulting income to the department/organization. It should be interesting and written as a story and be brief.

Objectives

These should be succinctly stated and use clearly defined *SMART* goals.

Market analysis

What to include will depend on the type of proposal. A summary should be given of the political and economic context. Competition includes not only the competition of competing groups but also of competing technologies. This section should also include a 'SWOT' analysis, that is, summarize the Strengths, Weaknesses, Opportunities, and Threats to the organization or unit (see SWOT analysis, p. 152). It may be relevant to define the market in which you compete, highlight its size, anticipated growth, and your market share, and to describe the nature and distribution of your 'customers' and the competition:

• 'Customers' (who, where, why, when).
• Competition (who, where, size, market share, strengths/weaknesses).

Benefits

This section should clearly identify the benefit against the alternative of doing nothing. Benefits should be quantified in both clinical quality and financial terms, where possible. Benefits to patients, staff, the organization, and the wider healthcare system should be considered.

Business concept

A detailed account of the proposed services should be provided. A cost–benefit analysis of the proposed investment should also be included. If there are different options these can be described here. The impact on the wider healthcare and possibly social care systems may be considered in order to put the change in context and to understand its full impact.

Options appraisal

Discuss alternative models of the proposed service, but importantly with the options, include the option of doing nothing.

Operations and management

This should highlight the unique operational and management aspects of the service. For example, how and where the staff delivers services and if the unit or organization is superior in its performance benchmarks when compared with other units or organizations. This section should include the impact on support services (e.g. X-ray, reception, pharmacy) and other clinical teams or organizations (e.g. primary care, social care), if there are any, and how you have engaged them so far.

Financial plan

Project revenue and expenses of the new service plus any savings. What will be the costs—the start-up cost, the cost of running the business, and additional sources of funds, including loan options?

Implementation plan

State your timescales and benchmarks, which not only show that you have carefully planned the steps of your proposal, but also help with any subsequent monitoring. This section should also include resource requirements from other departments and services and illustrate how you will work with them.

For some tips for success, see Box 2.13.

Box 2.13 Tips for success

- Do not attempt to do this alone.
- Seek out the finance director of the department/organization early in the process, plus key stakeholders in other organizations affected.
- Seek any relevant internal guidance and templates as they differ from place to place.
- Ensure the plan covers all the key questions tailored to the project and only keep if relevant.
- Ensure preparation of the plan is interdisciplinary, between the different clinical and management/financial stakeholders—your partners will have complementary skills.
- Ideally one person will lead on writing the plan, but with review and input from others.
- Identify who has financial skills.
- Clinicians will identify clinical priorities, opportunities, and risks.
- Consider the wider policy background of your plan (e.g. a plan should include the affordability and attractiveness of proposals to commissioners).
- Consider whether your proposal has any political implications that might attract the attention of your local authority and involve them.

Signposting

British Heart Foundation. *Business Case Toolkit*. [online] Available at: https://www.bhf.org.uk/for-professionals/healthcare-professionals/resources-for-your-role/business-case-toolkit (accessed 3/10/2021).

NHS Health at Work Network. *Business Planning Resources*. [online] Available at: https://www.nhshealthatwork.co.uk/business-plan-resources.asp (accessed 3/10/2021).

Further reading

Galloway, M. (2004). Best practice guideline: writing a business case for service development in pathology. *Journal of Clinical Pathology*, 57(4), 337–343. doi:10.1136/jcp.2003.012518

Jazayeri, A. and Park, K.T. (2019). How to write an effective business plan in medicine. *Gastroenterology*, 156(5), 1243–1247. https://doi:10.1053/j.gastro.2019.03.003

Leading for quality and safety

Introduction

Quality and safety of healthcare was once a given—now it is seen as a challenging endeavour, given the growing complexity of clinical care, as well as the way healthcare is delivered. Enabling the delivery of high-quality care and the proactive management of risk to prevent adverse events and harm is the responsibility of every leader, whether clinical or managerial.

Quality can broadly be defined as the degree of excellence of something, as compared to things of a similar kind. It is a comparator and is measurable against a standard. High-quality healthcare is defined into seven domains (Box 3.1).

Box 3.1 Seven domains of high-quality healthcare

Safe care is care that is free from avoidable harm. The World Health Organization defines patient safety as 'the prevention of errors and adverse effects to patients associated with health care'. It represents the practice, process, method, system, and science of reducing avoidable harm resulting from errors and adverse events.

Timely care is care that is delivered when it is needed and indicated without delay.

Effective care is evidence based and standardized (where scientific evidence and best practice standards exist). It represents the right care for the right patient, first time every time.

Efficient care is free from waste (cost, time, resources, consumables, procedures, medications, etc.), and strives to optimize value.

Equitable care offers fair allocation of and access to healthcare resources depending on individual patient need, irrespective of race, age, sex/gender, ethnicity, income, geographic location, or any other potential discriminator.

Sustainable care is future-proofed, environmentally friendly, and is reasonably resourced in the context of all societal needs.

Person-centred care (PCC) is enabling, personalized, coordinated, and delivered consistently with dignity, compassion, and respect. The term 'person-centred' also incorporates the human side of care provision. This proposes that clinicians be afforded the opportunity to realize meaning, purpose, and joy in their work to provide higher-quality care. This domain surrounds all the other domains.

The quality system has core values of kindness, compassion, respect, integrated and holistic care, and coproduction. Leadership for quality and safety is transparent and open to all as indicated in Fig. 3.1.

Quality in healthcare can be categorized into three phases, as indicated in Fig. 3.2 (Lachman et al., 2021). All are essential for high-quality outcomes.

Quality first started with the development of standards and then regulation. Best practice evidence-based standards and guidelines are an essential tool for optimizing high-quality and safe care. It is desirable for all patients and clinicians to plan and provide care, in keeping with the most up-to-date scientific evidence base.

The working realities of many healthcare environments, where clinical contact takes place in addition to resource constraints, may result in

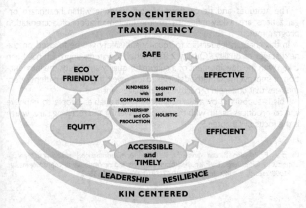

Fig. 3.1 The quality system.

Reproduced under Creative Commons Attribution License from Lachman, P., Batalden, P., and Vanhaecht, K. (2021). A multidimensional quality model: an opportunity for patients, their kin, healthcare providers and professionals to coproduce health. *F1000Research*, 9, 1140. https://doi.org/10.12688/f1000research.26368.2

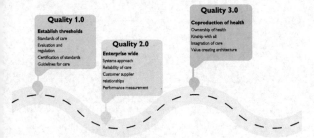

Fig. 3.2 Stages of quality in healthcare.

challenges to their application. Therefore, it is essential that standards and guidelines are contextualized and designed to be operable. This can be achieved through co-design and iterative testing with relevant clinicians and patients.

Regulation is the management of complex systems according to a set of rules and trends. Accreditation is concerned with the external assessment of organizations against designed, pre-approved standards. Regulation and accreditation provide for the application, inspection, and assurance of minimum standards to try to ensure patient safety. They represent a form of quality control.

Regulation and accreditation systems vary in their approach to engagement with care professionals, structures, and systems from very intermittent to almost continuous, and from oversight to actively supportive.

The attitudes and perceptions of staff working within healthcare organizations are a key influence on the implementation of accreditation programmes.

In this chapter, leadership for quality and safety will be focused on the next stages of quality, 'Quality 2.0', in which a systems approach has been taken with the development of a culture for quality and safety, the introduction of improvement methodologies to improve care, and the patient safety theories that underpin proactive risk management.

This is supported by a learning system that enables people to improve and co-produces health with the people delivering and receiving care, which is the focus of Chapter 5.

Reference

Lachman, P., Batalden, P., and Vanhaecht, K. (2021). A multidimensional quality model: an opportunity for patients, their kin, healthcare providers and professionals to coproduce health. *F1000Research*, 9, 1140. https://doi:10.12688/f1000research.26368.2

Developing a quality and safety culture

What is a quality and safety culture?

Culture is manifested as the shared values, practices, attitudes, and goals that characterize an organization. Healthcare organizations in which quality is a priority focus on building a culture of patient safety. They value a culture of safety as core to how they do their work and care for patients. They use practical safety tools and approaches to optimize safety across all facets of care.

Why is it important?

There are many studies and reports that demonstrate that failure in healthcare systems and processes is usually underpinned by a culture that does not place the quality and safety of health and healthcare at the core of all activities. Likewise, safe and high-reliability organizations and teams demonstrate a culture that is facilitative of safe behaviour and actions within a learning environment.

What's the theory?

Healthcare organizations that value a quality and safety culture engender the attitude in all staff that safety is paramount. These organizations build and learn continuously, working towards the organizational goal of measurably safer care. An example is the Cincinnati Children's Hospital Medical Centre which states that 'Safety is central to delivering the best-in-class outcomes we are committed to and is a fundamental right of the parents who bring their children to us for care' (https://www.cincinnatichildrens.org/).

A just culture recognizes wider design, organization, and systems causes for adverse events and unsafe care. This type of culture promotes psychological safety and creates greater opportunity to learn from the complexities of harm so that similar events can be prevented from recurring in future. It is the opposite to a blame culture, which seeks to hold individuals accountable for errors that occur. A blame culture can disincentivize adverse harm recognition and open disclosure, as punitive action may ensue.

How does this work in practice?

There are many actions one can take as a leader to develop safe behaviour and actions within a learning system that facilitates the culture that enables all to learn and continually improve. Examples of actions include the following:

- Walk the walk with safety walk-rounds to hear what is happening on the frontline.
- Create a learning reporting system in real time so that processes can be improved.
- Study what works well as well as what does not.
- Learn from and celebrate success and excellence.
- Develop safety huddles to be aware of safety and quality issues.
- Measure performance and learn (see Measuring system performance, p. 103).
- Involve patients and their families in co-designing the solutions (see Measuring person-centred care, p. 139).

- Introduce simulation to ensure clinical teams are able to react in a predictable way when required (see Introduction to simulation, p. 193).

Successful clinical leaders have the state of mind in which work is about quality and safety while we care for people.

Signposting

American College of Healthcare Executives and IHI/NPSF Lucian Leape Institute (2017). *Leading a Culture of Safety: A Blueprint for Success.* Boston, MA: American College of Healthcare Executives and Institute for Healthcare Improvement. Available at: http://www.ihi.org/resources/Pages/Publications/Leading-a-Culture-of-Safety-A-Blueprint-for-Success.aspx (accessed 19 July 2022).

Health and Safety Executive (2016). *Quality and Safety Walk-Rounds Toolkit.* [online] Available at: https://www.hse.ie/eng/about/who/qid/governancequality/qswalkrounds/quality-and-safety-walk-rounds-a-co-designed-approach-toolkit-and-case-study-report.pdf (accessed 19 July 2022).

The Kings Fund (2017). *Making the Case for Quality Improvement.* [online] The King's Fund. Available at: https://www.kingsfund.org.uk/publications/making-case-quality-improvement (accessed 19 July 2022).

Further reading

Dixon-Woods, M., Baker, R., Charles, K., et al. (2013). Culture and behaviour in the English National Health Service: overview of lessons from a large multimethod study. *BMJ Quality & Safety,* 23(2), 106–115. doi:10.1136/bmjqs-2013-001947

Mannion, R. and Davies, H. (2018). Understanding organisational culture for healthcare quality improvement. *BMJ,* 363(363), k4907. doi:10.1136/bmj.k4907

National Advisory Group on the Safety of Patients in England (2013). A Promise to Learn – A Commitment to Act: Improving the Safety of Patients in England. London: HMSO. Available at: https://assets.publishing.service.gov.uk/government/uploads/system/uploads/attachment_data/file/226703/Berwick_Report.pdf accessed 19 July 2022.

West, M.A., Topakas, A., and Dawson, J.F. (2014). Climate and culture for health care performance. In: B. Schneider and K.M. Barbera (eds) *The Oxford Handbook of Organisational Climate and Culture* (pp. 335–359). Oxford: Oxford University Press.

Understanding the system with improvement science

What is a healthcare system?

A clinical leader needs to understand the wider context within which work is undertaken. The healthcare system is a collection of interacting and inter-related entities (people, machinery, data, processes) organized around the common purpose of providing health and delivering healthcare. The way the health system is designed and how it works will determine the out-comes achieved. The systems approach to health studies how the different elements within the health system interact to produce outcomes, both de-sired and undesired. In highly complex systems, this offers an integrated perspective to allow us to assess how to improve the way component parts work and interact to achieve the outcomes.

Why is it important?

The original model for healthcare was linear with an interaction between a caregiver or clinician and a person/patient. As diagnoses and treat-ments became available, healthcare was organized into defined structures in primary, secondary, and tertiary care, each becoming more complex. Healthcare is now regarded to be a complex adaptive system which is composed of many parts that need to interact to achieve a desired out-come. To achieve safe, quality care, understanding how the system works is the first step to take.

What is the theory?

In 1986, Joseph Juran proposed a quality management trilogy for achieving high quality in industry. This can be applied to any work system:
- *Planning* quality by design. This requires an assessment of the system and what is needed for high-quality, safe services.
- *Control* of quality during ongoing operations, through regulation and measurement of the process.
- *Improvement* of outcomes by continuously improving quality.

Planning and control are often recognized as core management functions. Meaningful improvement requires effective leadership, as this third element of the trilogy inherently requires change.

Many quality improvement approaches are derived from the work of W. Edwards Deming. Deming's 'System of Profound or Improvement Knowledge' proposes a comprehensive framework through which complex quality problems can be better understood and solved for the purpose of improvement. It is composed of the four components or lenses through which a leader can analyse a system (Box 3.2).

Box 3.2 The lenses of profound knowledge
- An appreciation of a *system* (i.e. thinking about systems of care).
- An understanding of *psychology* (i.e. how humans behave).
- Knowledge of *variation* (i.e. in the processes to achieve outcomes).
- The theory of *knowledge* (i.e. epistemology and how change is made).

Appreciation of how the system works

For a clinical leader, the concept of a clinical microsystem is useful to understand where improvement can take place. The clinical microsystem is composed of patients and the healthcare team comprising doctors, nurses, and allied health professionals, in differing combinations (Fig. 3.3).

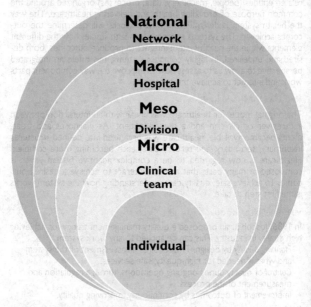

Fig. 3.3 Healthcare as a system (Dartmouth Institute).

For example, to achieve good outcomes for a person who has been referred to hospital (the macrosystem) for treatment of a stroke, different microsystems will need to interact to achieve rapid assessment and the desired outcome (e.g. reception, triage, radiology, neurology, etc.). The goal is to maximize the output of the system, rather than the output of each of its individual components.

Each clinical microsystem can be a powerful unit of quality improvement. Members of the microsystem have the most granular knowledge of how clinical processes work, how care is co-produced between fellow professionals and patients, and consequently are best placed to generate effective, workable, and meaningful improvements in quality and safety. Frontline ownership of improvement can be achieved if clinical leadership at the microsystem level is leading the changes required, rather than these being imposed.

To achieve this one should ask five key questions in real time (quality planning) so that one can continually assess how the microsystem is functioning (quality control) and how to improve (Table 3.1).

Table 3.1 The five Ps

Purpose	What is the purpose or stated aim of the clinical microsystem and do all share this purpose?
	This requires all members of the team to agree as to the purpose of the work
Patients	Who are the patients, what do they think of the service, and what is their experience?
	The patients may not be the people defined in the purpose, e.g. if there are outliers
	One also needs to understand the behaviour of patients to achieve outcomes
Professionals	Who are the members of the microsystem and what are their skills and needs, and views about the service?
	This includes all members of the team especially trainees who are rotating through the service. One also needs to understand the behaviour of healthcare workers to achieve outcomes
Processes	How are outcomes achieved—i.e. how is work done, is it standardized or is there variation?
	The team needs to analyse how work is done rather than how it is thought to happen, e.g. follow the guidelines
Patterns	How is performance measured over time?
	Does the team measure variation in the process and the outcomes achieved in real time to allow for improvement to be planned

Adapted from the Dartmouth Institute.

Understanding human behaviour—psychology

Human behaviour is a key element of change and an understanding of the belief and attitudes of team members is essential for a clinical leader. It is also important for managing the behaviour of patients when they are asked to implement change. The trans-theoretical model (Table 3.2) recognizes that individuals fall on a spectrum in relation to change. As a leader for quality and safety, being aware of what stage a stakeholder is at, in relation to change, can help understand whether they may be supportive, ambivalent, or resistant to change, and aid in planning how to incrementally build change-momentum and so improve quality and safety.

Table 3.2 Stages of change model (Prochaska and DiClemente)

Stage	Description
Pre-contemplation	Not considering change
Contemplation	Considering change in the future
Preparation	Recognize there is a problem and considering possible change
Action	Undertaking change
Maintenance	Sustaining the gains made from the change by monitoring and adjusting as needed
Relapse	Possible regress to previous behaviour

Change requires motivation and Maslow proposed a hierarchy of needs to explain the drivers for human motivation. This theory suggests that for somebody to strive to reach a higher level in the hierarchy, their more basic needs, at least partially, must be met first. The foundation of needs are the basic requirements for living and for safety. Once these are achieved, then a sense of belonging and achievement are possible (Fig. 3.4).

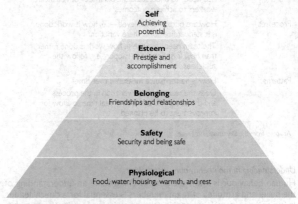

Self
Achieving
potential

Esteem
Prestige and
accomplishment

Belonging
Friendships and relationships

Safety
Security and being safe

Physiological
Food, water, housing, warmth, and rest

Fig. 3.4 Maslow's hierarchy of needs.

This is essential when building psychological safety. This will allow those being led to keep their focus on the higher purpose and goal of improving quality and safety. The creation of an environment in which everyone can strive for full self-actualization can both boost resilience and reconnect professionals with the meaning of their work.

Knowledge of variation

A feature of the way we do work is that variation is inherent in all processes. The study of variation allows the clinical leader to identify opportunities for improvement. Leading for quality and safety requires a basic understanding of variation, and particularly the difference between common cause and special cause variation (Table 3.3) (see Statistical process control charts, p. 106). This is the 'P' for patterns in the five Ps model.

Table 3.3 Differences between common and special type variation

Variation type	Characteristics	Example
Common cause	Produced by processes in a stable system Predictable	In a fully staffed and usually booked outpatient clinic, patients will expect to wait between 10 and 40 minutes to see a doctor
Special cause	Produced by extraordinary circumstances impacting the system and/or its processes Unpredictable	On one day, two doctors are delayed by an emergency on the ward and all patients wait for over an hour to be seen

Recognizing and understanding these two types of variation allows leaders to better understand system performance and to tailor quality and safety improvement interventions more appropriately. A key consideration here is recognizing that every system is designed to achieve precisely the results that it achieves. Asking a system to work harder is unlikely to produce real, sustainable, and measurable improvement. However, by disrupting and re-designing a system, it is possible to produce positive special cause variation and a new way of working to achieve genuine improvement.

Theory of knowledge to understand change

This lens alludes to epistemology and how people relate to, and value, knowledge. It focuses on how we achieve change and acknowledges the importance of belief in, and ownership over work, and the wider contextual reality within which we work (see Improvement methods, p. 76, and Chapter 6).

How does this work in practice?

See Box 3.3.

Box 3.3 Theory of knowledge in practice

Operation on time

A consultant general surgeon in a hospital grew frustrated that her operating list always started late. As a result, her last case, an ill patient having fasted all day, often had their procedure cancelled. She resolved to try to improve this problem using a quality improvement approach.

Building the will to change—psychology

She started by asking those involved in providing care in the operating theatre about their experiences, what they thought was working well and what they believed could be improved. This engagement included patients, the anaesthetic team, nurse managers, theatre nurses, porters, and administrative staff. Through these conversations, she realized that many others were as frustrated as she was by the current situation. She aimed to allow people to move from their basic needs to that of achievement, by moving them from pre-contemplation of change to planning and action.

Understanding the process in the systems

She undertook to understand the journey of the patient from how each procedure was booked, to discharge, including preoperative assessment, admission to the hospital, transport of the patient, pre-procedure care, operation theatre and staff preparation, anaesthesia, surgical site preparation, surgery itself, and post-procedure care.

She first imagined how these processes worked and then began to discuss each step in detail with those involved. From this, she realized that the process she imagined was very different to the work being done. She also recognized that she would need support and help from individuals and teams involved in every step of the process to remove waste to improve the theatre start time.

Measuring variation

With staff involved in each step, she started to measure separate parts of the process, in addition to the delay in theatre start time each day. This allowed everyone to see where delays were occurring and to appreciate both normal and common cause variation in the process. She excluded any special causes so that the team could concentrate on the common cause that were amenable to change.

Testing and implementing change—theory of knowledge

Patients and those most closely involved in areas where delays occurred were then invited to propose and test changes, with broad support from all groups involved in providing surgical care. As all these relatively small process improvements added up, more and more staff became actively involved. Once the operating list began to start on time, further procedures did not require cancellation, other than in exceptional circumstances. Though rare, these exceptional circumstances are now seen as a learning opportunity for every member of the wider surgical team to improve continuously.

Further reading

Batalden, P.B. and Davidoff, F. (2007). What is 'quality improvement' and how can it transform healthcare? *Quality and Safety in Health Care*, 16(1), 2–3. doi:10.1136/qshc.2006.022046

Godfrey, M.M., Foster, T., Johnson, J.K., et al. (2017). *Quality by Design: A Clinical Microsystems Approach*. Hoboken, NJ: John Wiley & Sons, Inc.

Kaplan, G., Bo-Linn, G., Carayon, P., et al. (2013). Bringing a systems approach to health. *NAM Perspectives*, 3(7). https://doi:10.31478/201307a

Mohr, J.J. (2002). Improving safety on the front lines: the role of clinical microsystems. *Quality and Safety in Health Care*, 11(1), 45–50. doi:10.1136/qhc.11.1.45

Royal Academy of Engineering (2017). *Engineering Better Care: A Systems Approach to Health and Care Design and Continuous Improvement*. London: Royal Academy of Engineering. Available at: https://www.raeng.org.uk/publications/reports/engineering-better-care (accessed 3/10/2021).

Improvement methods

Why is it important?

The way the delivery of care is designed has been a major cause of adverse outcomes in global healthcare. According to the World Health Organization, as many as four in ten patients are harmed in primary and outpatient healthcare. Up to 80% of harm is preventable. In Organisation for Economic Co-operation and Development (OECD) countries, 15% of total hospital activity and expenditure is a direct result of adverse events.

By leading for quality improvement and patient safety, there can be significant improvement to patient care and outcomes. Aiming for higher quality and safer care can result in ill health being managed more quickly, with greater competence, humanity, and without unnecessarily wasting resources. For individual patients, care can be reoriented around what really matters to that person, while clinicians can both reconnect with joy and purpose in their work and achieve higher levels of personal growth and fulfilment.

What is the theory and method?

Batalden and Davidoff (2007) specified that quality improvement requires a combined effort to make the changes that will lead to better patient outcomes (health), better system performance (care), and better professional development (learning). A leader who wants to continually improve must identify how the system is working and then analyse the causes of variation in performance. This will allow the development of an improvement programme based on continual measurement. There are five key steps to take:

1. Identifying variation in the process

Processes are the steps required to achieve an outcome. They have purposes and functions of their own but cannot work entirely by themselves. Process mapping is a method of visualizing all the activities and tasks of a process and how they interact with one another. The process map captures how the process works. It demonstrates the actual process rather than how it is presumed to operate, that is, 'work as done' as opposed to 'work as imagined' (see Process mapping, p. 153 for how to study a process).

Once the process has been mapped, one can look for variation, inefficiencies and duplication, unsafe steps, as well as unnecessary variation. Bottlenecks in processes which cause delays throughout the system are identified where a queue forms behind a step in the process. There is often more than one bottleneck in a process. The time to complete a process can have a significant impact on clinical outcomes. For example, for a patient suffering with a thrombotic stroke, the symptom onset to treatment time is critical. After identifying the bottleneck, steps can be taken to alleviate it, by rerouting work, finding ways of reducing delays at the bottleneck, and speeding up flow through this step.

2. Analysing problems using root cause analysis

For effective quality improvement to be implemented, one must understand the causes of the identified problem. Root cause analysis (RCA) describes a wide range of approaches, tools, and techniques that are used to uncover causes of problems. The benefit of a RCA is that it allows for better understanding of the causes of a problem and facilitates the development of solutions. As part of this approach one can use the 'five whys' to determine a problem's root cause (see Five whys, p. 156).

3. Analysis of variation using fishbone cause and effect

The fishbone diagram (also known as the Ishikawa diagram or cause-and-effect diagram) is a tool which helps to visually display the many potential causes of a specific problem or effect and enables diagnosis of a problem before starting the improvement process (see Fishbone diagram, p. 157).

4. Measurement for improvement

A leader needs to continually measure how the system is performing and whether improvement is required. Measurement also can be used to provide evidence of variation, to influence behaviour, and to provide an understanding of the process. Measurement for quality and safety improvement differs in purpose from measurement for research and audit. Measurement for research is designed to establish what is *possible*. Measurement for audit is designed to establish what is *actual*. Measurement for improvement is designed to assist in closing the gap between what is possible and what is actual (also known as the 'know-do' gap).

A clinical leader needs to understand the different types of measures to effect change. When measuring for the goal of improvement, these can then be categorized as any one of the following three types of measures: outcome, process, and balancing (Table 3.4).

Table 3.4 Types of measures for improvement

Measure type	Description	Examples
Outcome	The measure that describes what happens to the patient or staff member—overall system performance or aim of improvement	For hypertension: average blood pressure
		For access: number of days to first appointment
		For critical care: intensive care unit per cent unadjusted mortality
		For medication systems: adverse drug events per 1000 doses
Process	Elemental processes or components of the overall system which contribute to how the overall system performs	For hypertension: percentage of patients who had 24-hour ambulatory blood pressure monitoring in the past year
		For access: average daily clinician hours available for appointments
		For critical care: percentage of patients with intentional grounding completed on schedule
		For medication systems: number of nurse administration interruptions

(Continued)

Table 3.4 (*Contd.*)

Measure type	Description	Examples
Balancing	Other consequences of change to the system which can be positive or negative knock-on effects	For hypertension: number of myocardial infarctions prevented For access: waiting list size For critical care: intensive care unit bed days For medication systems: deaths due to medication error

Measures should have a clear and concise operational definition to establish an agreed and valid means of quantifying the variable in question. These definitions should be drawn up and agreed by all stakeholders involved, to ensure measurement is effective in achieving its purpose (Box 3.4).

Box 3.4 Summary of measurement for improvement

Getting started—measurement for improvement
1. Involve those affected in designing the measures.
2. Make the data collection as easy as possible.
3. Keep measurement intervals short (ideally no longer than 1–2 weeks apart).
4. Ensure you have baseline data to start with.
5. Plot your median with the baseline data initially.

Then
6. Confirm data collection method.
7. Collect data.
8. Analyse data and understand what the data says—it will tell a story.
9. Make change based on the data.

Repeat the cycle as continuous improvement.

Effective measurement for quality and safety is a dynamic and continuous endeavour. Traditional static, before-and-after approaches to data measurement and display are limited in their ability to influence behaviour on an ongoing basis and do not allow as broad or as early an understanding of variation in data over time, especially under conditions of change. Dynamic measurement using run charts and statistical process control (SPC) charts allows the effects of change to be evaluated and acted upon continuously (see Run chart rules, p. 104, and Statistical process control charts, p. 106).

Practical approaches to generating change
A clinical leader should know how to improve care and there are several methods one can use in improvement to test changes. As a leader for change, one needs to know about the one best for your context. The Model for Improvement, developed by Associates in Process Improvement (Fig. 3.5), provides a practical framework for improvement. It aims to operationalize one's theory with three core questions and then to test change ideas on a small and safe scale. This allows iterative learning, continuous

Model for Improvement

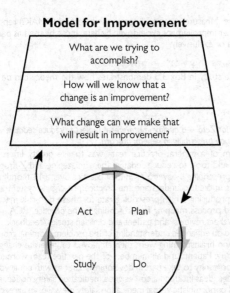

What are we trying to accomplish?

How will we know that a change is an improvement?

What change can we make that will result in improvement?

Act   Plan

Study   Do

Fig. 3.5 The Model for Improvement.
Reproduced with permission from Associates in Process Improvement, www.apiweb.org

honing of change strategy, and the intrinsic embedding of incremental change. This approach facilitates the solving of large and complex problems, through many small and workable changes, executed by those working within the system.

The Plan–Do–Study–Act (PDSA) cycle is used to test changes in real-world settings. The PDSA cycle is an easy-to-understand, structured approach for making small incremental changes to a system and for determining if that specific change is an improvement, and is refined at short intervals (daily or weekly) (see Assessing the need for change, p. 151).

Other practical frameworks for quality improvement deployed in healthcare settings include Lean and Six Sigma.

* Lean deploys standardized methodologies and tools to continuously improve quality through the elimination of waste. The core principle of Lean is that each step in the process must add value to the process and hence the outcome.
* Six Sigma uses a more data-driven approach to improve quality by eliminating defects and reducing variation, measuring using SPC charts (see Run chart rules, p. 104, and Statistical process control charts, p. 106).

- Define, Measure, Analyse, Improve, and Control (DMAIC) represents another improvement cycle driven by data. It can be used as part of Six Sigma or exclusively.

How does this work in practice?

The case study in Box 3.5 demonstrates how the theory can be put into action.

Box 3.5 A quality improvement project in action

'Zzz is for Zero'—a quality improvement project to reduce sedative medication prescribing in general practice

The aim of a general practice team was to use quality improvement theory and tools to reduce sedative (benzodiazepine and Z-drug) medication prescribing by over 50% in their practice over a 12-month period.

Tools utilized to understand the practice prescribing system and why it was producing a high prescribing rate for these high-risk medications included process mapping for prescribing in the practice, RCA, in-depth patient chart reviews, and patient and clinician stories/feedback.

Based on enhanced understanding of the problem, nominal group technique and brainstorming were then employed to generate change ideas for testing. Patients and all members of the practice team were afforded the opportunity to take part in developing solutions with equal voice.

Change ideas included a co-designed medication safety notice, a standardized opportunistic verbal medication safety message, an agreed clinical practice guideline on sedative medication prescribing, and a standardized approach to sleep hygiene resources. These change ideas were themselves iteratively tested and improved using PDSA cycles.

Baseline prescribing and improvement was measured in total milligrams of common sedative medications prescribed by the practice each week.

Signposting

NHS England (2017). The How to Guide for Measurement in Improvement. [online] Available at: https://www.england.nhs.uk/improvement-hub/wp-content/uploads/sites/44/2017/11/How-to-Guide-for-Measurement-for-Improvement.pdf (accessed 3/10/2021).

Reference

Batalden, P.B. and Davidoff, F. (2007). What is 'quality improvement' and how can it transform healthcare? Quality and Safety in Health Care, 16(1), 2–3. doi:10.1136/qshc.2006.022046

Further reading

Perla, R.J., Provost, L.P., and Murray, S.K. (2011). The run chart: a simple analytical tool for learning from variation in healthcare processes. BMJ Quality & Safety, 20(1), 46–51. doi:10.1136/bmjqs.2009.037895

Provost, L.P. and Murray, S.K. (2011). The Health Care Data Guide: Learning from Data for Improvement. San Francisco, CA: Jossey-Bass.

Patient safety theories and methods

Why is it important?

Patient safety has become one of the major public health issues due to the increasing complexity of healthcare and the growing awareness that in most cases harm and adverse events can be prevented. Up to 15% of all people are harmed while in hospital and more in the community. The World Health Organization has designated the decade 2021–2030 as the decade of patient safety and has published a world action plan.

An adverse event is often the result of an error (Table 3.5).

Table 3.5 Error and adverse events

Error	The failure of a planned action to be completed as intended (i.e. error of execution) or the use of a wrong plan to achieve an aim (i.e. error of planning). An error may be an act of commission or an act of omission
Adverse event	Results in unintended harm to the patient by an act of commission or omission rather than by the underlying disease or condition of the patient

Patient safety science aims to apply scientific knowledge and theory into practical methods to decrease harm.

What is the theory?

As a clinical leader, one needs to understand the theories of patient safety to be able to proactively manage risk.

Swiss cheese model

James Reason proposed the Swiss cheese model of system accidents. This model describes how both *active failures* (unsafe acts committed by people) and *latent conditions* (system design flaws with the potential to result in fallibility on the part of the system) contribute to harm. The model proposes a dynamic interplay between these two types of factors whereby each can create holes in the defensive layers (technological, procedural, personal, and administrative) of a system. When these holes temporarily align, harm can occur. While the holes in Swiss cheese are static, these holes are dynamically opening, closing, and changing shape in the complex adaptive system that is healthcare.

Human factors and ergonomics

(See Patient safety and human factors learning, p. 190.)

Human factors and ergonomics (HFE) is an evidence-based discipline that uses a design-driven systems approach to achieve two closely related outcomes of performance and well-being. A failure to apply human factors principles is believed to be a key contributor to 70–80% of adverse events.

The principles and practices of HFE focus on optimizing human performance through better understanding the behaviour of individuals, and their interactions with each other and with their environment. Through applying this approach, errors can be reduced.

HFE draws from the areas of psychology, anatomy and physiology, social sciences, engineering, design, and organizational management to design environments and processes that make it easier for healthcare professionals to provide safe care. The Systems Engineering Initiative for Patient Safety (SEIPS) assesses how the different elements of the work system are interacting (i.e. the culture, environment, people, tasks, and technology). These in turn develop the processes that result in either safe or unsafe outcomes/health.

A key part of HFE is the development of the cognitive aspects of safety in the form of situation awareness. Strong team-based situation awareness requires clear communication and can be enhanced using a structured communication at a clinical huddle or handover meeting and a structured communication checklist (e.g. SBAR or I-PASS).

Reliability
(See Innovation versus change, p. 147.)

Reliability theory draws on the key attributes of highly reliable and safe industries (nuclear power, aviation, military) and applies these principles to healthcare. Table 3.6 lists the attributes of high-reliability teams.

Table 3.6 Attributes of high-reliability teams

Attribute	Practical action	Healthcare example
Preoccupation with failure	Look for errors and encourage reporting to learn	Small errors before they become adverse events, e.g. prescribing errors
Sensitivity to operations	Share situation awareness	Knowing how the teams are working in real time using tools such as surgical timeout and checklists
Deference to expertise	Communication from and decision-making at frontline	Nurse recognizes incorrectly prescribed medication and does not administer
Reluctance to simplify	Create more complete pictures of situations	Planning patient care using a multidisciplinary approach and do not have linear thinking
Commitment to resilience	Ability to identify, control, and recover from the unexpected	Resuscitation training and practising urgent case-based scenarios
		Learning from what is working and what is not

Resilience or 'Safety 2'
Safety 2 defines safety as the ability to succeed under varying conditions, in contrast to the traditional view of safety as being conspicuous in its absence, with resulting harm. It recognizes a growing body of work aiming

to generate safer care, through learning from care processes and systems, which for the most part work well. The key is to study how work is done rather than as it is imagined on protocols and guidelines. This will assist in building resilience and learning from what works, as safety is seen as being able to adapt constantly to changing circumstances. This will lead to pro-active planning to be safe using humans as a resource rather than as the problem.

How does this work in practice?

See Box 3.6.

Box 3.6 Improving patient safety through enhanced situation awareness

Situation Awareness for Everyone (S.A.F.E.) toolkit

The S.A.F.E. toolkit aims to improve patient safety through enhanced situation awareness among healthcare teams. Team-based situation awareness is augmented using structured safety huddles. A huddle is a brief team meeting to share understanding of what has happened, what is happening, and what will happen in the future for individual patients and their care.

The purpose of the huddle is to assess and identify patients who may deteriorate, to mitigate active risk and to escalate observation or care where necessary. For the huddle to be effective, every member of the team must feel psychologically safe to contribute (see Developing a safe learning system, p. 85).

This can be achieved by ensuring that every opinion offered is recognized and is seen to count, that all views are respected, that input is sought from patients and their family members, and that hierarchy in running the huddle is rotated. Patients often identified as needing a closer watch ('watchers') at and after the huddle include those where a family member has raised a concern, on high-risk medication, who have a rising early warning score, where there is more than one clinical team involved, on an unusual ward, or about whom the nurse feels 'they are just not right'.

The S.A.F.E. approach results in earlier recognition of deteriorating patients, improved team communication, and less avoidable patient harm (see https://www.rcpch.ac.uk/resources/situation-awareness-everyone-safe-toolkit-introduction).

Signposting

NHS England (n.d.). SBAR Communcation Tool. [online] Available https://www.england.nhs.uk/wp-content/uploads/2021/03/qsir-sbar-communication-tool.pdf. accessed 9/09/2022
Patient Safety Learning. [online] Available at: https://www.patientsafetylearning.org/

Further reading

Chartered Institute of Ergonomics and Human Factors (CIEHF) (2018). *Human Factors for Health & Social Care (White Paper)*. Birmingham: CIEHF. Available at: https://www.lboro.ac.uk/media/media/schoolanddepartments/design-and-creative-arts/downloads/CIEHF-2018-White-Paper_Human%20Factors-in-Health-Social-Care.pdf (accessed 19/07/2022)
Holden, R.J. and Carayon, P. (2021). SEIPS 101 and seven simple SEIPS tools. *BMJ Quality & Safety*, 30(11), 901–910. doi:10.1136/bmjqs-2020-012538

Holden, R.J., Carayon, P., Gurses, A.P., et al. (2013). SEIPS 2.0: a human factors framework for studying and improving the work of healthcare professionals and patients. *Ergonomics*, 56(11), 1669–1686. doi:10.1080/00140139.2013.838643

Hollnagel, E., Wears, R.L., and Braithwaite, J. (2015). *From Safety-I to Safety-II: A White Paper*. [online] Available at: https://www.england.nhs.uk/signuptosafety/wp-content/uploads/sites/16/2015/10/safety-1-safety-2-whte-papr.pdf (accessed 19/072022).

Shahian, D. (2021). I-PASS handover system: a decade of evidence demands action. *BMJ Quality & Safety*, p.bmjqs-2021-013314. doi:10.1136/bmjqs-2021-013314.

The Health Foundation (2013). *The Measurement and Monitoring of Safety in Healthcare*. London: The Health Foundation. Available at: https://www.health.org.uk/publications/the-measurement-and-monitoring-of-safety (accessed 3/10/2021).

Vincent, C. and Amalberti, R. (2016). *Safer Healthcare*. Cham: Springer International Publishing. doi:10.1007/978-3-319-25559-0

Wilson, K.A. (2005). Promoting health care safety through training high reliability teams. *Quality and Safety in Health Care*, 14(4), 303–309. doi:10.1136/qshc.2004.010090

Developing a safe learning system

Why is it important?

Leadership is the essential ingredient to facilitate safety and quality in healthcare. One of the fundamental roles of leadership is to develop a milieu within which people can feel safe, so that they can be safe, and then act safely. Leaders cannot assume this will happen and need to have a form of collaborative and dispersed leadership—knowing when to lead and when not to.

What is the theory?

Psychological safety can be defined as being able to show and employ oneself without fear of negative consequences of self-image, status, or career. To achieve safe and high-quality care, it is incumbent on all to lead by establishing a psychologically safe environment where all team members can realize their full potential and value to the improvement process. Three steps can build psychological safety (Fig. 3.6).

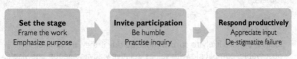

Fig. 3.6 Practical steps for building psychological safety.

Psychological safety is often threatened in healthcare by cynicism, disguised as realism, arrogance dressed up as authoritative knowledge, and callousness portrayed as the thick skin of experience. In destroying psychological safety, these behaviours greatly limit creative thinking, daring, curiosity, eagerness to question, compassion, and connection, core mindsets for effective quality improvement. If people have meaning and purpose in their work, and then feel valued, the chances of their being safe will be enhanced.

Leading for change

(See Leading for change, p. 11, Measuring system performance, p. 103, and Types of change, p. 145.)

Leading a quality improvement project or a clinical team requires you to bring others on board. To engage the team, the tips shown in Box 3.7 can be useful:

In Chapter 6, tools such as stakeholder maps and communication plans are discussed.

Box 3.7 Tips for leading for change

- Create an urgency for change by using data and stories.
- Look for the intrinsic motivators. Point the listener towards the 'attractors' for them (i.e. consider taking time to ask questions first to find out what these may be).
- Appeal to extrinsic motivators (i.e. the core healthcare values of care and compassion).
- Balance optimism and critical thinking; be positive and considered.
- Be energetic and resourceful as a 'can-do attitude' goes a long way and energy can attract others.
- Tailor your leadership style to your audience as an effective pitch for a chief financial officer may differ to that for a care assistant.
- Consider a 'tagline' that can be repeated during the pitch with a few words that will stick.
- Make it safe for team members to challenge and ask questions.
- As a leader, continually practise and improve how you engage with others.

Testing change ideas

- Ideas are more likely to spread more quickly if they are simple, observable, compatible with values, relatively advantageous, and viable.
- Quality improvement works by dividing problems into their smallest possible components and exploring change through small incremental 'testing' of ideas. Testing occurs using a PDSA cycle (see Learning, p. 79).
- The results of these tests can be to adopt, adapt, or abandon a small change. As opposed to larger-scale implementation of change, testing can happen more safely for those potentially affected by it, and without fear of failure for those seeking to generate improvement.
- When you add these small tests together, their sum can be a significant improvement that has been built by everyone who has taken part in a test.
- The concept of testing also affords the opportunity to start before anyone is 'ready', thus facilitating rapid learning and progress.

Resistance to change

(See Leading for change, p. 11, and Winning hearts and minds, p. 166.)
- Change can be a daunting and challenging experience for many with psychological and physiological resistance to change.
- Not everyone will embrace change at the same rate, but they are more likely to if they feel supported and are active participants, not merely passengers in the change journey.
- A clinical leader must recognize that there are both technical (the change itself) and social (emotional) challenges to improvement.
- To achieve this, a leader should unleash internal motivation for change, allow co-design and co-production of the solutions to be tested and implemented, and distribute power to the frontline clinical microsystem.

Signposting

Perlo, J., Balik, B., Swensen, S., et al. (2017). *IHI Framework for Improving Joy in Work*. IHI White Paper. Cambridge, MA: Institute for Healthcare Improvement. Available at: http://www.ihi.org/resour ces/Pages/IHIWhitePapers/Framework-Improving-Joy-in-Work.aspx (accessed 19/07/2022).

Further reading

Edmondson, A.C. (2018). *The Fearless Organization: Creating Psychological Safety in the Workplace for Learning, Innovation, and growth*. Hoboken, NJ: John Wiley & Sons, Inc.

Heifetz, R.A., Linsky, M., and Harvard Business Review Press (2017). *Leadership on the Line: Staying Alive Through the Dangers of Change*. Boston, MA: Harvard Business Review Press.

Hilton, K. and Anderson, A. (2018). *IHI Psychology of Change Framework to Advance and Sustain Improvement*. Boston, MA: Institute for Healthcare Improvement. Available at: http://www.ihi.org/resources/Pages/IHIWhitePapers/IHI-Psychology-of-Change-Framework.aspx (accessed 19/07/2022).

Patients or people as partners for quality and safety

Why is it important?

Positive patient or person experience is associated with increased clinical effectiveness and fewer adverse events. Achieving partnership with patients and their family members can make care safer by regarding patients as persons or people receiving care.. At the level of the individual, patients can play an active role in co-producing safer care, through enhancing the interdependent relationship between clinician and patient.

In addition to the benefits for individual patients, many organizations invite the participation of patients and family members at governance level, for their valuable insights as people with direct care experience and for their non-healthcare-related expertise. This can be a particularly enlightening and effective strategy to improve accountability for patient safety at all levels. Quality 3.0 requires a partnership between the healthcare system and the people whom we call patients. This partnership can co-design and deliver the quality and safety that is required.

What is the theory?

Coproduction

(See Co-production, p. 132.)

A clinical leader can co-produce solutions with both staff and patients. Co-production has been defined as 'the interdependent work of users and professionals to design, create, develop, deliver, assess, and improve the relationships and actions that contribute to the health of individuals and populations'.

Box 3.8 Practical examples of involving patients in leadership

Governance

- Patients and representatives can be part of the governance structures in hospitals, to be able to set policy.
- All board meetings should start with a patient and staff narrative so that the board can make decisions in the light of their lived experience.

Quality improvement programmes and projects

- Patients or patient representatives should be part of the design and implementation of improvement programmes and projects.
- Patients and families can determine what should be measured—that is, what really matters to them.

Building resilience

- Patient experience can be used to build resilience within the system as they know how the process works.
- Add a patient story of good care at every ward round as well as care that can be improved.

Learning

- Patients and families can be part of clinical incident investigations as equal participants.

Involving patients and their family members as active partners in all stages of healthcare quality and safety generation is an extremely effective way to gain a deeper understanding of health and care from the perspective of the service user. This facilitates an improvement approach that can resonate with true professional purpose and a committed partnership with shared accountability for delivering higher-quality and safer care based on what matters to people receiving care (Box 3.8).

Signposting

NHS England (2021). *Framework for Involving Patients in Patient Safety*. [online] Available at: https://www.england.nhs.uk/publication/framework-for-involving-patients-in-patient-safety/ (accessed 19/07/2022).

Patient Safety Learning. [online] Available at: https://www.patientsafetylearning.org/ (accessed 19/07/2022).

Further reading

Batalden, M., Batalden, P., Margolis, P., et al. (2015). Coproduction of healthcare service. *BMJ Quality & Safety*, 25(7), 509–517. doi:10.1136/bmjqs-2015-004315

Doyle, C., Lennox, L., and Bell, D. (2013). A systematic review of evidence on the links between patient experience and clinical safety and effectiveness. *BMJ Open*, 3(1). doi:10.1136/bmjopen-2012-001570

O'Hara, J.K., Aase, K., and Waring, J. (2018). Scaffolding our systems? Patients and families 'reaching in' as a source of healthcare resilience. *BMJ Quality & Safety*, 28(1), 3–6. doi:10.1136/bmjqs-2018-008216

The Health Foundation (2014). *Patient-Centred Care Made Simple*. London: The Health Foundation. Available at: https://www.health.org.uk/publications/person-centred-care-made-simple (accessed 19/07/2022).

Wiig, S., Hibbert, P.D., and Braithwaite, J. (2020). The patient died: what about involvement in the investigation process? *International Journal for Quality in Health Care*, 32(5), 342–346. doi:10.1093/intqhc/mzaa034

Leadership for improving outcomes

Introduction

All healthcare workers want to provide high-quality care for their patients, but how do we know when this has been achieved? On the other hand, how can we tell when care has perhaps been suboptimal?

What constitutes good-quality care can be difficult to define, particularly as outcomes for care must be defined for all conditions and treatments that are offered in clinical practice. This can be challenging. For example, could (or should) the same metrics be used to assess the success of treatment for depression as are used to assess the success of a hospital admission for pneumonia?

For clinicians to lead the debate and progress on improving care and improving outcomes for the population they serve, they must first understand how healthcare is funded and assessed. To this end, the first half of this chapter covers the important topics of commissioning, benchmarking, quality, and outcomes.

The second half of this chapter will outline how we define good quality healthcare, by focusing on what constitutes 'value' for patients and describing what is needed to construct a value-based healthcare system, drawing on the work of Kotter and others.

Healthcare systems around the world are increasingly struggling with the costs of providing good healthcare. All healthcare practitioners need to own financial responsibility for service provision. For the aspiring leader, a sound knowledge of how to produce good overall outcomes—both for patients and healthcare systems—is now more vital than ever before.

Commissioning

What is commissioning?

Commissioning is the process by which services are designed and funded.

Why is this important?

There are numerous ways to pay for health services. The focus in this chapter will be on how it has been achieved in England and Wales. The concepts of the purchaser–provider split resulted in commissioning and has become an important process in developing and tendering for services. Clinicians are involved in delivering commissioned services, setting the case for new services, and can influence commissioning planning and decisions for the population of patients that they care for.

What is the theory?

Definitions and descriptions of commissioning are varied and complex. The one used here is the purchase of health services by an organization or group of clinicians acting on behalf of a population, based on health needs. There are two distinct roles in the commissioning process:
- Planning and designing services, understanding the needs of a population.
- Deciding who should provide services and how much they should be paid to do so.

Commissioning cycle

The commissioning cycle has similar components to the PDSA cycle used in quality improvement (Box 4.1 and Fig. 4.1).

Box 4.1 Commissioning cycle

Analyse (act)
- Examining the needs and expectations of service users.
- Consider existing legislation and guidance.
- Reviewing existing services and resources.
- Agree outcomes for any proposed services.

Plan
- Identify gaps in current services.
- Consider how to develop the service, what additional resources need to be considered.

Do
- Deliver service to achieve outcomes.
- Quality assurance.

Review (study)
- Impact of the service.
- How to improve.

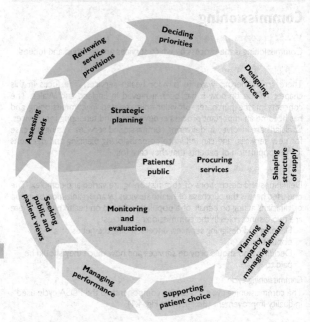

Fig. 4.1 Commissioning cycle.
Reproduced from The Kings Fund and NHS England under Open Government Licence.

How does this work in practice?

Many factors can affect commissioning models. These include whether the service has been commissioned previously, the market in which services exist, and what competition is present competing for funding. Relationships, both past and present, between commissioners and provider organizations influence the climate for negotiations.

Commissioners may use different processes in different areas or for different types of services, and clarity should be sought in clarifying these processes. For example, commissioning may be linked to a payment for results incentive process.

Where a commissioning process has been undertaken, criticisms can arise where unrealistic expectations have been set for a service which are difficult to achieve. Once a service is set up, commissioners have relatively little control over the outcome or operation of a service.

The role of the service user is often under-represented in the commissioning process, and the opinions and viewpoints of commissioners and providers can dominate the commissioning process. Commissioning should consider the social determinants of health to ensure equity of service delivery and to enhance equity of outcomes.

For some tips for success, see Box 4.2.

Box 4.2 Tips for success
- Get to know your commissioners and initiate conversations regarding services to help build a collaborative approach to commissioning.
- Understand the cost benefits of services.
- Involve service users in designing services and developing priorities for commissioning.
- Always consider the equity of the service commissioned and whether it addresses the social determinants of health.

Further reading

Robertson, R. and Ewbank, L. (2020). *Thinking Differently about Commissioning: Learning from New Approaches to Local Planning*. London: The Kings Fund. Available at: https://www.kingsfund.org.uk/publications/thinking-differently-commissioning (accessed 3/10/2021).

Benchmarking

What is benchmarking?

Benchmarking is the process of regularly comparing services with best practice and/or peers.

Why is this important?

Many organizations have the same aims to deliver high-quality care to their patients, some with greater success than others.

What is the theory?

The main principles of benchmarking are to maintain quality, achieve customer satisfaction, and to strive for continuous improvement (Box 4.3).

Each participant can compare and improve their own performance with a clearer understanding of competitors and service user needs. Benchmarking allows for the more rapid spread of innovation.

Box 4.3 Types of benchmarking

Internal benchmarking
- Can occur when one part of an organization has a better performance indicator than other areas.
- Other departments can learn how this improvement in performance was achieved.
- Benefits of being quick to identify and disseminate, as well as being a readily available resource within an organization.

External benchmarking or external evaluation
- May be competitive, comparing a service against a direct comparator (e.g. another hospital).
- Functional benchmarking can occur when organizations compare themselves against business and services operating in similar areas or similar activities (e.g. hospitals have compared to service industries).

Aspirational benchmarking
Healthcare organizations can benchmark against aspirational outcomes, for example, to mirror clinical trial and evidence-based outcomes.

How does this work in practice?

Benchmarking requires substantial investment in terms of time, cost, and resources. Benchmarking tools and databases exist to simplify the process but only add to highlight some of the challenges of benchmarking. Rather than knowing that there is a difference between organizations (e.g. methicillin-resistant *Staphylococcus aureus* acquisition in a hospital), it is beneficial to understand how better performance is different in context, such as resource availability, local factors, and population factors (Box 4.4). This should be considered when undertaking benchmarking against other organizations.

Box 4.4 Examples of metrics for benchmarking

- Measures of productivity markers.
- Quality measures, time, and cost.
- Clinical outcome measures.
- Patient satisfaction and experience measures.
- Analysis of unwarranted variation.
- Measures for cost benefit of processes.
- Benchmarking on integration of care.
- Workforce optimization.
- Governance.
- Readiness for crises.

Accreditation by an external evaluation body can provide a hospital with regular assessment against sets of standards. These are then the foundation for a programme of continual improvement.

For some tips for success, see Box 4.5.

Box 4.5 Tips for success

- Consider a range of metrics including patient outcomes in benchmarking.
- Be cautious to ensure outcome metrics are comparable, for example, different organizations may have differing recording processes.
- If you notice differences in performance between areas, spend time trying to understand how these occur, and in what circumstances the other service operates. What can you learn from them?
- Do not limit benchmarking comparisons to healthcare organizations.
- Consider what elements of your service may be being delivered by other organizations and look to learn from other industries.

How do you do this already?

Most services look to benchmark themselves, either internally on generic metrics or locally with similar services. This includes auditing against best practice. If you have ever done an audit of your service (e.g. following national guidelines), you are carrying out a form of benchmarking.

Signposting

NHS Benchmarking Network. [online] Available at: https://www.nhsbenchmarking.nhs.uk/ (accessed 3/10/2021).

Royal College of Nursing (2017). *Understanding Benchmarking*. London: Royal College of Nursing. Available at: https://www.rcn.org.uk/professional-development/publications/pub-006333#detailTab (accessed 3/10/2021).

Quality and outcomes

What is quality?

Quality in healthcare is about providing patients with the care that they need, when they need it, in a safe, affordable, and effective way (see Chapter 3). The Institute of Medicine defined quality in healthcare as 'the degree to which health services for individuals and populations increases the likelihood of desired health outcomes and are consistent with current professional knowledge'.

Why is this important?

As clinicians, we wish to provide a service of high quality. We must be confident that we can articulate what quality is, how to recognize and measure it, and how to continually improve it. It is important to recognize that other people may hold different views and definitions regarding quality, including patients.

What is the theory?

As noted in Chapter 3, the domains of quality are integrated and cross over into each other. With the advent of the climate change challenge, another domain is now considered to be essential. Sustainable care is future proofed, environmentally friendly, and is reasonably resourced, as compared to other societal needs. The quality of any service is affected by multiple factors, some which may be within our control as clinical leaders and some which may be outside direct control. When considering the quality of any service, care should be taken to understand which services, individuals, and factors contribute to the quality of care. Any intervention to improve quality should aim to focus on one of the domains of quality.

How does this work in practice?

The quality of a service can be viewed differently by managers, clinicians, and patients who may have different perspectives and expectations. To implement an improvement programme, one needs to demonstrate that there is a problem. This requires the study of the system and the processes in the system and measurement of the outputs or outcomes of the system.

Challenges include convincing people that there is a problem and a potential solution, whether there is a leadership focus on improvement, and being able to collect the data. There may be tribalism, professional rivalries, and the lack of staff engagement, all of which can make the improvement process difficult to implement. The use of an improvement method as described in Chapter 3 can alleviate these challenges.

For some tips for success, see Box 4.6.

Box 4.6 Tips for success

- Consider a broad approach to assessing the quality of your service within the domains of quality.
- Carefully plan what data is required to demonstrate the quality of the service, and which areas need improvement.
- Familiarize yourself with improvement methodology and consider tools available to approach quality improvement.

Further reading

Institute of Medicine (US) Committee on Quality of Health Care in America (2001). *Crossing the Quality Chasm: A New Health System for the 21st Century*. Washington, DC: National Academies Press.

Langley, G.E., Moen, R.D., Nolan, K.M., et al. (2009). *The Improvement Guide*, 2nd ed. San Francisco, CA: Jossey-Bass.

The Health Foundation (2021). *Quality Improvement Made Simple*. London: The Health Foundation. Available at: https://www.health.org.uk/publications/quality-improvement-made-simple (accessed 3/10/2021).

What is an outcome?

What are outcomes?

Outcome indicators are markers of the result of healthcare. Different groups may have different interests in different types of outcomes (e.g. mortality versus functional state).

Why is this important?

Outcomes are reported across a wide number of specialties. It is now expected that all specialties report their own outcomes, either as a peer review to commissioners or management, or to patients and their carers.

What is the theory?

Outcomes may exist for a range of elements of care, and many are indicators of care rather than endpoint outcomes. Donabedian proposed that structures and the processes within the structures produce the outcomes achieved, which are either desirable or undesirable. A study of the work system and its components will assist in understanding how outcomes are achieved.

The work system is composed of how the organization or team is structured. This is an interaction between culture (beliefs and attitudes), the tasks that need to be undertaken, the technology that is available to complete the tasks, the environment in which the work is done, how the work is organized, and the people involved in delivering and receiving the care. These all will interact to produce the processes of care, that is, how work is done to achieve outcomes.

Desirable outcomes depend on having the right structure and processes in place and as such must be used with an understanding of the environment in which care is being delivered. A balanced set of measures for all improvement includes a combination of outcome measures, process measures, and balancing measures (Boxes 4.7–4.9).

Box 4.7 Measures of structures or systems

These measure how the service is designed and take a system view, such as staffing, tools and equipment, environment and organizational or system design, and culture.

Examples
1. Culture surveys.
2. Equipment available.
3. Level of education and skills.
4. Staffing levels.

Box 4.8 Process measures

Process measures describe how care is delivered to patients and whether processes are performing as planned. They are most useful in chronic disease management and ambulatory care. Process measures focus on how care is delivered and can demonstrated unwarranted variation in delivery of care. They are often easy to interpret and allow for actions to be taken to improve the care delivered. Examples are:

Diabetes

Percentage of patients whose haemoglobin A1c level was measured twice in the past year; neuropathy testing in patients.

Populations

Screening programme being undertaken.

Access

Average daily clinician hours available for appointments.

Critical care

Percentage of patients with intentional grounding completed on schedule.

Box 4.9 Outcome measures

Outcomes are the result of healthcare, that is, what happens to the person receiving care.

- Population outcomes (e.g. cancer mortality, hospital admission rate).
- Clinical care outcomes (e.g. blood pressure control, readmission rates).
- Adverse events (e.g. drug administration error).
- Patient experience of care (e.g. patient experience survey feedback/complaints).
- Patient health and/or functional status.
- Patient-reported outcome measures (PROMs) and patient-reported experience measures (PREMs) (see Measuring person-centred care, p. 139).
- How does this impact patients, their health, or well-being? This feedback can be gained in a variety of ways: patient interviews, surveys, focus groups, observation, and complaints.
- How does the system impact the values of patients, their health, and well-being? What are the impacts on other stakeholders such as payers, employees, or the community?

Examples

- For hypertension: average blood pressure.
- For access: number of days to first appointment.
- For critical care: intensive care unit per cent unadjusted mortality.
- For medication systems: adverse drug events per 1000 doses.

How does this work in practice?

Outcome measures must be measured by condition, not procedure or intervention. They should reflect the full cycle of care for a condition and reflect the results most relevant to patients and consider the initial condition and risk factors, measured in a standardized manner. Box 4.10 describes some causes for variation.

Box 4.10 Causes for variation

Causes for variation in outcome measures
- Differences in patient type (e.g. comorbidity, severity).
- Impact of external factors (e.g. reliance on external services).
- Difficulties in measurement.
- Chance (influenced by the number of cases in a cohort).
- Differences in the quality of care.
- Unwarranted variation in the delivery of care.

Example: unilateral hip replacements in England

Since 2009, PROM data have been collected for unilateral hip replacement by the NHS. Prior to the operation, consent is obtained and the generic PROMs EQ-5D™ Index and EQ-VAS™, and specific condition PROM Oxford Hip Score completed. These data have been used by providers to identify areas where patients think they perform well, and where they can improve; by commissioners to identify and share areas of good practice and encourage improvement; and by service users to review the location they may wish to choose for their procedure if this is available.

For some tips for success, see Box 4.11.

Box 4.11 Tips for success

- Ensure outcome measure is relevant to clinical work being undertaken.
- Be conscious of potential causes for variation within outcome and quality measures.
- Recognize the patient's viewpoint, and outcome and quality measures that are important to the patient.
- When choosing or designing a tool to characterize PROM and PREM data for a particular condition, it is advisable for the evaluation measure to be co-designed to have meaning for patients and clinicians/services.
- The tools chosen must be validated to have any meaning.

Further reading

Donabedian, A. (1988). The quality of care. *JAMA*, 260(12), 1743–1748. doi:10.1001/jama.1988.03410120089033

EuroQol Group (2021). ED-5Q-5L™. [online] Available at: https://euroqol.org/eq-5d-instruments/eq-5d-5l-about/ (accessed 13/1/2021).

Holden, R.J., Carayon, P., Gurses, A.P., et al. (2013). SEIPS 2.0: a human factors framework for studying and improving the work of healthcare professionals and patients. *Ergonomics*, 56(11), 1669–1686. doi:10.1080/00140139.2013.838643

Kingsley, C. and Patel, S. (2017). Patient-reported outcome measures and patient-reported experience measures. *BJA Education*, 17(4), 137–144. doi:10.1093/bjaed/mkw060

Nelson, E.C., Eftimovska, E., Lind, C., et al. (2015). Patient reported outcome measures in practice. *BMJ*, 350, g7818–g7818. doi:10.1136/bmj.g7818

Weldring, T. and Smith, S.M.S. (2013). Patient-reported outcomes (PROs) and patient-reported outcome measures (PROMs). *Health Services Insights*, 6, 61–68. doi:10.4137/hsi.s11093

Measuring system performance

What is performance?

Performance of a system (see Chapter 3) is described by the level to which a service is delivering on several predefined performance indicators. These indicators can be considered individually and in aggregate to give an overall picture.

Why do we measure performance?

Measuring performance is important to demonstrate the effectiveness of a service and to review whether improvement is required.

Why is this important?

Quality is dependent on how the complex system interacts to produce the clinical outcome. System outcomes can be viewed in terms of the cost, the clinical outcome, and from lenses of the domains of quality. Organizations, clinical bodies, commissioners, and patients want to be able to review performance data for a service in order to determine whether it is safe, effective, and delivering good value for money, and to be able to contextualize it in other demands on budgets. Demonstrating positive performances in key indicators will reassure internal organizational monitoring and external scrutiny that a commissioned service is delivering what it is intended to, and to identify areas for improvement.

What is the theory?

Main purposes of measuring performance

Performance measurement describes the present, that is, how an intervention in a specified group of patients produces the outcomes for a specific treatment or management plan. It can also measure improvement in outcomes following an improvement intervention (assuming all other factors remain stable), and provide a comparison of the quality of care delivered to different groups.

Considerations when measuring performance

As with any measure, there is a risk of confounding factors that impact the outcome measure. Care must be taken when deciding which service or intervention is to be evaluated. The types of measure (process, structure, outcome) must be decided.

In deciding on measures, consider the target audience as patient groups will have a different requirement from a measure compared to clinicians, who may have a different requirement from an organizational board of directors or from commissioners. The intended effect of the measure must be recognized as outcome measures can be powerful motivators for change (e.g. an improvement in outcomes following a pilot intervention to secure longer-term resources).

Problems when measuring performance

The challenges of measurement include inadequate information systems, not enough or incorrect data collected, waiting for the perfect data system, and the tendency to have too many measures which are confusing. The complexity of healthcare delivery (e.g. multiagency care across a wide geographical area) may make data comparisons challenging, and data collected may be interpreted as to its intent (e.g. when stating a case for investment), as opposed to clinical outcome.

How does this work in practice?

The use of time series analysis is the best way to demonstrate improvement and quality over time. These are also known as 'run charts'. A 'run' is one or more consecutive data points on either side of the median line. The median is the number found at the exact middle of the set of values it is not skewed by outlying data and therefore represents a fairer reflection of usual system performance. Run charts are sufficient for most quality and safety improvement work.

A run chart is developed as follows:

- Decide the variable you are measuring.
- Collect baseline data for the variable you are measuring (outcome, process, or balancing measure).
- Draw x- and y-axes.
- Label y-axis with measurement (e.g. day, per cent, rate, number).
- Label x-axis with value being measured and scale (usually time scale).
- Plot data points.
- Draw a line connecting the points.
- Calculate the median and draw it on the chart.

An example of a run chart structure is shown in Fig. 4.2.

Additional information can be added to the run chart. It may be appropriate to add a goal or target line. Annotation of unusual events, changes that are being tested, or other pertinent information can also be added to the chart to 'tell the story'. Annotations enhance communication and learning from run charts, for example, to find out what impact the changes have had on the system or process.

To know that the changes made to a system are resulting in improvement, and that the data being measured are not merely trending in a particular direction by chance, statistical rules can be applied.

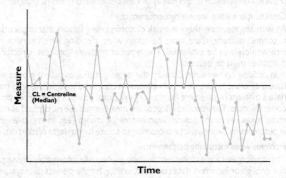

Fig. 4.2 Run chart outline.
Reproduced with permission from East London NHS Foundation Trust.

Run chart rules

Run charts have rules that can inform a leader and the team whether there is improvement or not (Fig. 4.3). A run chart should include at least 15 or more data points before applying any of the run chart rules.

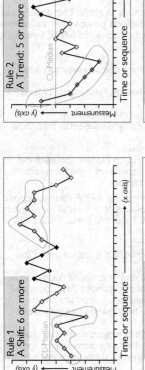

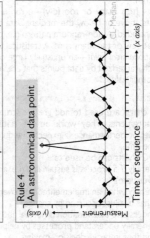

Rule 1
A Shift: 6 or more

Measurement (y axis)

CL Median

Time or sequence (x axis)

Rule 2
A Trend: 5 or more

Measurement (y axis)

CL Median

Time or sequence (x axis)

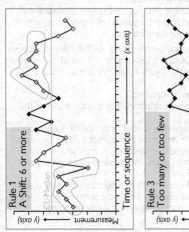

Rule 3
Too many or too few

Measurement (y axis)

CL Median

Data line crosses median once so only two runs, too few runs according to statistical table.

Time or sequence (x axis)

Rule 4
An astronomical data point

Measurement (y axis)

CL Median

Time or sequence (x axis)

Fig. 4.3 Run chart rules.
Reproduced with permission from East London NHS Foundation Trust.

Shift—a shift on a run chart is six or more consecutive points, either all above or all below the median. A shift is likely to be attributable to a change made and suggests non-random variation. Values that fall on the median neither add to, nor break a shift. Therefore, skip values that fall on the median and continue counting.

Trend—a trend on a run chart is five or more consecutive points, all going up or all going down. If the value of two or more successive points is the same, ignore one of the points when counting (these do not make or break a trend).

Run (too many or too few)—a run is one or more consecutive data points above or below the median. Data points that fall on the median are not included. A non-random pattern (i.e. change has occurred) is indicated by too few or too many runs. A statistical table is required to interpret runs.

Astronomical point—an unusually large or small number: an outlier. They are characterized by data points that are very different from all, or most of, the other values.

Statistical process control charts

SPC charts are used to add greater scrutiny to results from performance measurements. They work on the statistical principle that variation in events or performance is expected and occurs within defined limits most of the time.

SPC charts can be used to:
- identify if a process is sustainable (i.e. are your improvements sustaining over time)
- identify when an implemented improvement has changed a process (i.e. it has not just occurred by chance)
- understand that variation is normal and to help reduce it
- generally understand processes by helping to make better predictions and thus improve decision-making
- recognize abnormalities within processes
- prove or disprove assumptions and (mis)conceptions about services
- drive improvement—used to test the stability of a process prior to redesign work, such as demand and capacity.

Like run charts, data are plotted over time (Fig. 4.4). A mean as opposed to a median is used with upper and lower control limits of two standard deviations above and below the mean. These incorporate around 99% of all data.

Two types of variation can be identified:
- *Special causes variation* requires closer analysis as it is not part of the normal process.
- *Common cause variation* within the control limits may be due to normal variation, but there are circumstances that prompt a closer look at the system. Wide variation suggests an inefficient system, and one may want to review the system in place. The following situations are of relevance:
  - Any point outside of the control limits suggests a significant change.
  - A run of seven points all above or below the centre (mean) line (or all decreasing or increasing) suggests a significant change is

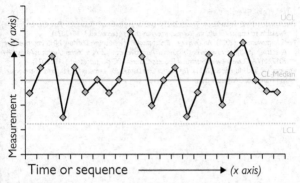

Fig. 4.4 SPC chart.

Reproduced with permission from East London NHS Foundation Trust.

- underway—this may be expected (e.g. following an improvement programme).
- Any unusual patterns or trends within the control limits (e.g. cyclical peaks and troughs in performance).

There are several differen t types of SPC chart that can be used, and more details on these are in signposted resources.

For some tips for success, see Box 4.12.

Box 4.12 Tips for success

- Explore what data your organization routinely collects, or what is able to be pulled from existing datasets (be cautious about data quality).
- There may be people in your organization who are skilled in data analysis and SPC charts—get to know them and ask for their support in reviewing performance (in hospitals typically such skills can be found in quality or improvement teams or in hospital informatics departments).

How do you do this already?

Most departments present data about their activity or performance, with increasing use of SPC charts in clinical settings. Review how your department reviews its performance —are the measures used an accurate reflection of the service and is the evidence presented robust?

Signposting

NHS England (2022). *Statistical Process Control Tool*. [online] Available at: https://www.england.nhs. uk/statistical-process-control-tool/ (accessed 20/07/2022).

NHS Institute for Innovation and Improvement (2017). *A Guide to Creating and Interpreting Run and Control Charts*. [online] Available at: https://www.england.nhs.uk/improvement-hub/wp-cont ent/uploads/sites/44/2017/11/A-guide-to-creating-and-interpreting-run-and-control-charts. pdf / (accessed 20/07/2022).

Further reading

East London NHS Foundation Trust (2021). *Quality Improvement Resources: Run Charts.* [online] Available at: https://qi.elft.nhs.uk/resource/run-charts/ (accessed 3/10/2021).

NHS Improvement (2011). *An Overview of Statistical Process Control.* London: NHS Improvement. Available at: https://www.england.nhs.uk/improvement-hub/wp-content/uploads/sites/44/2017/11/An-Overview-of-Statistical-Process-Control-SPC.pdf (accessed 3/10/2021).

Provost, L.P. and Murray, S. (2011). *The Health Care Data Guide: Learning from Data for Improvement.* San Francisco, CA: Jossey-Bass.

Creating a value-based healthcare system

What is value-based healthcare?

Porter and Lee (2013) describe value-based healthcare as having one overarching goal: to create value for patients. Value is defined as the outcomes that matter for patients and the cost to achieve those outcomes. They propose that healthcare should not be organized around the provider of care but rather around the patient and their needs for the condition to be managed.

There are six elements to this system which are described in detail in the following sections:

1. Organization in integrated practice units (IPUs).
2. Measurement of outcomes and costs for every patient.
3. Moving to bundled payments for care cycles.
4. Integration of care delivery across separate facilities.
5. Expansion of excellent facilities across geography.
6. Building an enabling information technology (IT) platform.
7. Financial incentives and outcomes.

Each of these stages interrelate to all other in a continuous and dynamic way, allowing for flexibility and improvement within the system, each aspect taking account of other aspects. In the following sections, we will further elaborate on the features of a value-based healthcare system.

Signposting

Harvard Business School (2021). Value-based healthcare website and resources. [online] Available at: https://www.isc.hbs.edu/health-care/value-based-health-care/Pages/default.aspx (accessed 3/10/2021).

Reference

Porter, M. and Lee, T. (2013). The strategy that will fix health care. *Harvard Business Review*. Available at: https://hbr.org/2013/10/the-strategy-that-will-fix-health-care (accessed 20/07/2022).

Further reading

Porter, M.E. and Lee, T.H. (2018). What 21st century health care should learn from 20th century business. *NEJM Catalyst*, 4(5). doi:10.1056/CAT.18.0098

Integrated practice units

What is an integrated practice unit?
Key attributes of an IPU:

- IPUs are organized around a patient's medical condition, or set of closely related conditions.
- A dedicated multidisciplinary team is formed who devote the majority of their time to the condition.
- All providers involved are members of or are affiliated with a common organizational unit.
- An IPU takes responsibility for the full cycle of care for the condition, including outpatient, inpatient, and rehabilitative care as well as supporting services (e.g. nutritional needs, social work).
- IPUs incorporate patient education, engagement, and follow-up as integral to care.
- IPUs use a single administrative and scheduling structure, and are co-located in dedicated facilities.

- Care is led by a care manager and physician team 'captain' who oversee each patient's care process.
- IPUs measure outcomes, costs, and processes for each patient using a common information platform.
- Members of the IPU function as a team, meeting formally and informally on a regular basis to discuss patients, processes, and results.
- Importantly, the IPU accepts joint accountability for outcomes and costs.

Why is this important?

Traditionally, hospital departments are split according to medical specialties such as cardiology, surgery, oncology, etc. However, this is both extremely inconvenient for patients and a highly inefficient way of treating patients with several comorbidities. For example, a person with diabetes may need to see an endocrinologist, vascular surgeon, cardiologist, and ophthalmologist for various different complications of the disease, necessitating multiple trips to various departments.

What is the theory?

IPUs are multidisciplinary, and focused on a condition (e.g. rheumatoid arthritis, diabetes, renal failure), rather than a specialty. In this way, an IPU can be responsible for the full cycle of patient care. Patients benefit from a 'one-stop shop', and clinicians and other healthcare providers benefit from improved interactions with their colleagues.

How does this work in practice?

The IPU concept may be used to decrease readmissions in those patients at highest risk. Ideally, they should be across primary, secondary, and tertiary care so that admission to hospital is avoided. With the introduction of telemedicine, integration becomes essential.

These centres compare favourably with the inefficient sequential specialist patient care processes of earlier eras in several different domains; for example, staff learning has been enhanced, facilitated by the volume and concentrated focus of the units; multidisciplinary teamwork has improved; and overall better clinical outcomes have been noted (Box 4.13).

Box 4.13 IPUs in action

At the beginning of the 1990s, the University of Texas MD Anderson Cancer Center underwent a 5-year reorganization of outpatient care services, moving towards disease-specific IPUs. This transition towards multidisciplinary care required massive reorganization of staff, equipment, and facilities.

As a result, a typical MD Anderson care centre is now a high-volume, disease-specific platform for focused care, where specialist care for patients is performed by members of a dedicated team.

For some tips for success, see Box 4.14.

Box 4.14 Tips for success
(See Inter-professionalism, p. 179.)
• A successful IPU will define the disease condition(s) it wishes to treat and will work with others to ensure that holistic care can be provided for these condition(s).
• Teamwork and good communication are essential to link different facets of care. As much as possible, the team should be co-located.
• Importantly, the success of the IPU should be measured according to metrics that are relevant to the disease being treated; they should reflect an improvement in the overall state of the patient's condition.

Example
A diabetes IPU in north London provides several services based around the disease, including access to a diabetes nurse specialist, psychological assessment and intervention, dietician advice, podiatrist review, a joint kidney disease/diabetic clinic, and other counselling services.

This has occurred through partnership with a variety of providers, crossing organizational boundaries, with the aim that patients are at the centre of their care and see the correct professionals with the correct skillset at the correct time.

Measures of outcomes and costs
What do we mean by outcomes and costs?
While the concept of outcomes is highly familiar to healthcare providers, value-based healthcare stresses the importance of standardizing the way we define outcomes so that they are:
• patient focused, and
• comparable across different healthcare settings.

Similarly, the costs incurred to reach these outcomes can be determined in a number of ways; a traditional model may look only at the costs incurred to provide a service (e.g. fee for every MRI performed).

Why is this important?
Many hospitals and healthcare providers are already rewarded for their outcomes, but what has been missing in the past is how well the care delivered meets an individual patient's needs; for example, did the treatment delivered allow a patient to return to work or, in more severe cases, to care for themselves?

In a similar fashion, a standardized approach to costing allows better understanding of the link between individual patient outcomes and the costs incurred in reaching them.

What is the theory?
• An outcomes measure hierarchy can be used to measure outcomes. This incorporates values which are important to both healthcare providers and patients in combination.
• Tier 1 includes those that are most important, including survival and the degree of health or recovery obtained by the patient.

- Tier 2 includes other factors that, although important, are not as vital as those in tier 1, such as the time for recovery and return to other activities, and any disutility of care or treatment processes, such as delayed care or adverse effects from medication.
- Lastly, tier 3 outcomes look at other important factors, such as the sustainability of health (recurrences) or the long-term consequences of treatment.

How does this work in practice?

For outcomes, the International Consortium for Health Outcomes Measurement (ICHOM) focuses on measuring and reporting patient outcomes in a standardized way. The ICHOM works with physicians, outcomes researchers, and patient advocates to define standard sets of outcomes for a wide range of medical conditions such as cardiovascular and musculoskeletal disorders. The organization has worked with a variety of providers, both private and public, internationally, and provides a variety of case studies on its website demonstrating its methodology and approach.

Principles of measuring the cost of care

For costs, Porter and Lee (2013) have outlined the principles for measuring the cost of care as detailed in Box 4.15.

Box 4.15 Principles to measure cost

- Cost should be measured around the patient.
- Cost is not the charges billed or collected, but rather the actual expense of patient care.
- Cost should be aggregated over the full cycle of care for the patient's condition, rather than being collected for an individual department, procedure, consultation, or piece of equipment.
- Cost depends on the actual use of resources involved in a patient's care process (personnel, facilities, supplies), including:
  - the time devoted to each patient by these resources
  - the capacity cost of each resource
  - the support costs required for each patient-facing resource.

Measuring costs can start by using the management tool of process mapping, whereby each step of a patient's care pathway can be characterized and the costs associated with it quantified. Time-driven activity-based costing (TDABC) has become the gold standard approach to costing, and a comprehensive TDABC Project Support Pack is available free of charge from Harvard Business School (see 'Signposting').

Signposting

Harvard Business School (2020). *The Time-Drive Activity-Based Costing (TDABC) Project Starter Kit*. [online] Available at: https://www.isc.hbs.edu/Documents/pdf/2020_TDABC_Project_Starter_Kit.pdf (accessed 3/10/2021).

International Consortium for Health Outcomes Measurement (n.d.). *Resources*. [online] Available at: www.ichom.org (accessed 3/10/2021).

Reference

Porter, M. and Lee, T. (2013). The strategy that will fix health care. *Harvard Business Review*. Available at: https://hbr.org/2013/10/the-strategy-that-will-fix-health-care (accessed 20/07/2022).

Further reading

Porter, M. E., Larsson, S., and Lee, T. H. (2016). Standardizing patient outcomes measurement. *New England Journal of Medicine*, 374(6), 504–506. doi:10.1056/NEJMp1511701

Bundled payments for care cycles

What are bundled payments?

Bundled payments tie payments to overall care for a patient with a particular condition, and are aligned to things that the team can control. For acute medical conditions, a bundled payment covers the full care cycle, while for chronic conditions, the payment covers overall care over the course of a defined period of time such as a year. They may also cover primary or preventative care for defined patient populations (e.g. children).

Why are they important?

Two payment models are currently favoured in healthcare:

- *Global capitation*: in this model, a single payment is made to cover all of the patient's needs. Therefore, providers are incentivized to spend less, but not necessarily to improve outcomes or value.
- *Fee-for-service*: while this allows providers some control over the level of service they choose to provide, they remain unable to completely control overall costs or outcomes.

The deficiencies in these two models mean that an improved payment system is necessary to create true value for patients.

What is the theory?

By paying several different health providers simultaneously, they are encouraged to work together to improve costs, avoid duplication, and to improve quality and outcomes.

Although at first glance bundled payments may look similar to capitation payments as previously described, an important difference should be noted in that global capitation payments are generally made as an amount per patient to deliver services over a set period of time, whereas bundled payments are guaranteed each time an agreed bundle of care is delivered.

How does this work in practice?

Maternal care is a good example of bundled payment and many US obstetricians charge one flat-fee payment for all pre-delivery care and investigations, labour and delivery, and follow-up. A similar model is now in use in some areas of the UK, where 'pathway payments' are given to obstetric care providers, who are must also pay a secondary provider if they give some elements of care.

Alternatively, an orthopaedic procedure such as a knee replacement would not cover just the operation, but also the presurgical work-up, anaesthetist, the implant itself, and any postoperative tests, examinations, physiotherapy, or other rehabilitation required.

Bundled payments have been successfully adopted in several healthcare systems, including in Sweden, Germany, and the US. In the latter, bundled payments have become the norm for organ transplant care.

Further reading

Haas, D., Kaplan, R., Reid, D., et al. (2015). Getting bundled payments right in healthcare. *Harvard Business Review*. Available at: https://www.medtronic.com/content/dam/medtronic-com/global/Corporate/Initiatives/harvard-business-review/downloads/getting-bundled-payments-right-in-healthcare.pdf (accessed 3/10/2021).

OECD (2016). *Better Ways to Pay for Health Care*. OECD Health Policy Studies. Paris: OECD Publishing. doi:10.1787/9789264258211-en

Witkowski, M., Higgins, L., Warner, J., et al. (2013). How to design a bundled payment around value. *Harvard Business Review*. Available at: https://hbr.org/2013/10/how-to-design-a-bundled-payment-around-value (accessed 13/1/2021).

Integrated care delivery systems

What is integrated care?

Comprehensive healthcare is rarely provided at one location or site, particularly as the population continues to age and patients with multiple comorbidities become more common.

Although value-based healthcare suggests minimizing the impact of this problem through the establishment of IPUs (see Integrated practice units, p. 109), different IPUs may need to be run in different locations. Therefore, for a multisite healthcare system, knowing how to integrate care efficiently across locations is vital to create maximum healthcare value.

Why is integrated care important?

- When patient care is spread over different geographical locations, the risk of fragmented care and duplication of services is increased.
- As a result, patient health and satisfaction may be compromised, and costs may be inflated.

What is the theory?

- Integrating healthcare systems is a key priority in value-based healthcare. When services are not integrated it is possible for massive inefficiencies to exist (e.g. blood samples having to be routinely couriered from one site to another).
- A systematic review has shown that integrated care delivery systems have a positive effect on quality of care.

How does this work in practice?

Porter and Lee (2013) have identified four main areas that organizations must address in order to integrate care delivery systems.

1. Defining the scope of services

Providers determine which services they can realistically provide with high value, and which they may have to exit or partner with other organizations to provide. Service-line reporting may be helpful in this regard (Box 4.16).

2. Concentrating volumes in fewer locations

Although some have argued that providing services in local areas is most patient-friendly, Porter and Lee argue that this is a poor strategy for creating value. Certainly, for complex procedures, the relationship between procedural volumes and good patient outcomes provides a compelling argument for this approach. However, it may be that more routine, low-risk procedures can be successfully relocated to the community.

3. Choosing the right location for each service line

Many simple paediatric and surgical procedures, which are low risk and performed in high volume, may be best moved to community locations, freeing time in teaching hospitals for complex surgeries such as aortic reconstructive procedures.

4. Integrating care for patients across locations

While care should be directed by IPUs, the actual geographical location of services need not be fixed. However, care needs to be taken to try to maintain continuity of care through other mechanisms, such as using common treatment protocols and standardizing administrative procedures. In one example, use of integrated electronic health records helped to decrease office visits.

Box 4.16 Service-line management and reporting

Service-line management (SLM) was first introduced into healthcare in the 1980s in the US, and later developed by Monitor for NHS foundation trusts, to improve the way that healthcare is delivered.

SLM promotes the restructuring of health services into narrow business units (or 'service lines'), which are managed as distinct operational units, and which can be analysed for their ability to make or lose money. In doing so, clinical leaders within these service lines are empowered to manage services in a more cost-effective and sustainable way, and to reduce waste.

Service-line reporting is a crucial part of SLM and allows hospitals to improve their financial governance and efficiency by providing data on financial performance, activity, quality, and staffing. As a result, clinicians and managers can plan service activities, set objectives and targets, monitor their service's financial operational activity, and manage performance.

Signposting

NHS England Monitor (2009). *Service Line Management Collection*. [online] Available at: https://www.gov.uk/government/collections/service-line-management-an-approach-to-hospital-managment (accessed 20/07/2022).

Reference

Porter, M. and Lee, T. (2013). The strategy that will fix health care. *Harvard Business Review*. Available at: https://hbr.org/2013/10/the-strategy-that-will-fix-health-care (accessed 20/07/2022).

Further reading

Foot, C., Sonola, L., Maybin, J., et al. (2012). *Service-Line Management Can it Improve Quality and Efficiency?* [online] The Kings Fund. Available at: https://www.kingsfund.org.uk/sites/default/files/service-line-management-quality-efficiency-kings-fund-january2011.pdf (accessed 11/5/2022).

Gröne, O. and Garcia-Barbero, M. (2001). Integrated care. *International Journal of Integrated Care*, 1(2), e21. http://doi.org/10.5334/ijic.28

Hwang, W., Chang, J., LaClair, M., et al. (2013). Effects of integrated delivery system on cost and quality. *American Journal of Managed Care*, 19(5), e175–e184. Available at: https://www.ajmc.com/view/contributor-institutional-engagement-with-physicians-is-key-to-managing-cost-and-quality (accessed 3/10/2021).

Expanding geographic reach

What do we mean by expanding geographic reach?

For healthcare providers that provide exemplary care to patients, an opportunity exists to provide greater value by increasing the geographic locations at which this care is provided. This is particularly the case for tertiary and 'quaternary' centres—the latter is sometimes used to refer to advanced levels of medicine that are highly specialized, and which are usually only available in a few national or regional health centres.

What is the theory?
- If specialist hospitals wish to expand, constructing or purchasing another hospital outright is costly. Moreover, although such a move would likely increase volumes, costs and outcomes may suffer thereby worsening the value equation.
- Alternative models are therefore necessary, which allow providers to broaden their geographic scope, while maintaining the high standards of care that their service has become renowned for.

How does this work in practice?
Two main models are proposed, as shown in Table 4.1.

Table 4.1 Expanding reach

Model	Description	Example
Hub-and-spoke model for specialist centres	In this model, effective healthcare providers establish satellite units that are staffed—at least in part—by clinicians and other personnel from the parent organization, thus helping to standardize care across the organization	In the US, MD Anderson Cancer Center has four satellite centres in the greater Houston area that operate under the supervision of a 'hub' IPU. Of note, the cost of care at the satellite is substantially less
Clinical affiliation	This model involves IPUs partnering with local community organizations and using their facilities to provide care	The Cleveland Clinic's Heart & Vascular Institute works with several hospitals on the east coast of the US In the UK, Great Ormond Street Hospital holds several outreach clinics in other areas of the country providing, for example, specialist immunology care

Further reading

Elrod, J.K. and Fortenberry, J.L. (2017). The hub-and-spoke organization design: an avenue for serving patients well. *BMC Health Services Research*, 17(S1). doi:10.1186/s12913-017-2341-x

Building an enabling information technology platform

What is an enabling IT platform?
- IT systems in healthcare have become infamous for their complicated nature, lack of broad utility, and inability to communicate with other systems. Indeed, often IT platforms are seen to hinder—rather than enable—good care.

- An *enabling* IT platform plays a crucial role in value-based healthcare, in that it facilitates the strategy outlined previously, for example by ensuring that different hub and spoke centres communicate efficiently.

Why is this important?
- The inability of different IT platforms to communicate in the US costs billions of dollars each year.
- In the UK, the problems experienced by the NHS IT programme have had a significant impact on patient care as staff struggled to use the new systems.
- Written medical records are inefficient, to the extent that they may even impair clinical practice. For example, a patient's written medical file can only be accessed by one person in one place at any one time. Delays are incurred while patient notes are transferred from one healthcare provider to another.

How does this work in practice?
Porter and Lee (2013) list the key features of an effective IT platform:
- Centred on patients.
- Uses common data definitions.
- Encompasses all types of patient data.
- Medical record is accessible to all parties involved in care.
- The system includes templates and expert systems for each medical condition.
- The system architecture makes it easy to extract information.

At present, a multitude of different platforms exist, each with their relative strengths and weaknesses. For example, integration with mobile devices is prioritized more in some systems than others. Fortunately, the digital revolution has ensured that new providers are constantly emerging and challenging the status quo.

Reference

Porter, M. and Lee, T. (2013). The strategy that will fix health care. *Harvard Business Review*. Available at: https://hbr.org/2013/10/the-strategy-that-will-fix-health-care (accessed 9th September 2022).

Further reading

Chen, C., Garrido, T., Chock, D., et al. (2009). The Kaiser Permanente electronic health record: transforming and streamlining modalities of care. *Health Affairs*, 28(2), 323–333. doi:10.1377/hlthaff.28.2.323

Feeley, T.W., Landman, Z., and Porter, M.E. (2020). The agenda for the next generation of health care information technology. *NEJM Catalyst*, 1(3). doi:10.1056/cat.20.0132

Financial incentives and outcomes

What are financial incentives?
In the broadest sense, financial incentives describe how healthcare systems and providers are remunerated for the services that they perform. Currently, a wide variety of reimbursement models exist in healthcare systems around the world.

Why are they important?
- The two main contemporary models of financial reimbursement for healthcare provision mentioned previously (global capitalization and fee for service) are inadequate. For example, fees paid directly for services performed do not focus sufficiently on how the service influenced patient outcomes, and could even encourage overtesting.

- Alternatively, if a single payment is made to cover all of a patient's needs, providers may be tempted to cut costs, thereby negatively impacting care.

What is the theory?

- In keeping with the principles of value-based healthcare, in recent years several pay for performance (P4P) incentives have been introduced. For example, in the US, P4P initiatives are utilized by half of all commercial healthcare maintenance organizations, and are used in the payment of physicians, hospitals, and nursing homes. In the UK, almost 25% of primary care income comes from P4P incentives.
- Payment for performance rewards healthcare providers for reaching a predefined level of care, such as ensuring that the majority of patients in a primary care provider's practice have a blood pressure that is treated to within guidelines. Nonetheless, P4P has been criticized for having a limited impact on patient outcomes. Others argue that it is too soon to fully assess the overall impact of these measures, particularly in the treatment of chronic conditions such as heart disease and diabetes.

How does this work in practice?

- There is some evidence that P4P schemes can lead to a clinically significant reduction in mortality rates. In the advancing quality programme in North West England, providers were rewarded for being top performers in their area and for improving on their previous attainment. Overall, there was a clinically significant reduction in mortality for three of the five incentivized conditions, estimated to be the equivalent of 890 fewer deaths over 18 months.
- Due to their direct relationship with patient outcomes, it is likely that P4P initiatives will become increasingly popular over coming years. Mehrotra et al. (2010) have suggested seven key improvements to further increase the impact of P4P programmes, as shown in Table 4.2.

Table 4.2 Methods to increase the impact of P4P programmes

Current model	Suggested improvement
Incentive given as a lump sum	Divide the lump sum into a series of smaller incentive payments
Relative thresholds (e.g. top 25% of physicians)	Tiered absolute thresholds (e.g. 25%, 50%, 75%, 90%)
Long lag time between care and receipt of incentive	Shorten lag time to as short as possible
Use of withhold payments	Bonus payment or use of deposit contracts
Complex uncertain structure of programme (e.g. shared savings programme)	Simplify programme so that uncertainty is minimized
Incentive often given as an increase in fee schedule reimbursement	Decouple incentive payment so that it is given separately, consider a lottery
Monetary incentives	'In kind' incentives

From Mehrotra et al. (2010).

There remains a need for further research and evaluation of P4P systems. Evaluations have yielded mixed results, and caution should be exercised in interpreting data from different specialties and health systems. For example, a recent systematic review carried out on the Veterans Health Authority identified that P4P, which has been used in that system for many years, could have the unintended consequence to promote overtreatment (Kondo et al., 2018); similarly, ambiguous results have been found from systematic reviews in the UK (Kondo et al., 2016; Mandavia et al., 2017). Nonetheless it remains an important area of healthcare funding development and a lever for improvement.

Reference

Kondo, K.K., Damberg, C.L., Mendelson, A., et al. (2016). Implementation processes and pay for performance in healthcare: a systematic review. *Journal of General Internal Medicine*, 31(S1), 61–69. doi:10.1007/s11606-015-3567-0

Kondo, K.K., Wyse, J., Mendelson, A., et al. (2018). Pay-for-performance and veteran care in the VHA and the community: a systematic review. *Journal of General Internal Medicine*, 33(7), 1155–1166. doi:10.1007/s11606-018-4444-4

Mandavia, R., Mehta, N., Schilder, A., et al. (2017). Effectiveness of UK provider financial incentives on quality of care: a systematic review. *British Journal of General Practice*, 67(664), e800–e815. doi:10.3399/bjgp17x693149

Mehrotra, A., Sorbero, M.E.S., and Damberg, C.L. (2010). Using the lessons of behavioral economics to design more effective pay-for-performance programs. *American Journal of Managed Care*, 16(7), 497–503. Available at: https://www.ajmc.com/view/ajmc_10jul_mehrotra_497to503/ (accessed 20/07/2022).

Further reading

Mathes, T., Pieper, D., Morche, J., et al. (2019). Pay for performance for hospitals. *Cochrane Database of Systematic Reviews*, 7(7), CD011156. doi:10.1002/14651858.cd011156.pub2

Sutton, M., Nikolova, S., Boaden, R., et al. (2013). Reduced mortality with hospital pay for performance in England. *Obstetrical & Gynecological Survey*, 68(3), 187–189. doi:10.1097/01.ogx.0000428158.81933.54

Leadership for person-centred care

Introduction

Person-centred care (PCC) is a way of thinking that determines all the interactions one has with the person receiving care, as well as the person's family, kin, and community. In Chapter 3, the different levels of quality were introduced (Box 5.1).

Box 5.1 Levels of quality
- Quality 1.0: standards, regulation, accreditation, and certification.
- Quality 2.0: systems and reliability.
- Quality 3.0: co-production of health and value in partnership with people delivering and receiving care.

In this chapter, the focus will be on how to develop partnerships with the people receiving care, so that care is compassionate, kind, and respectful, as well as safe and effective. This implies that clinicians do not only focus on diagnosis and management of a disease, but rather treat patients as people who have lives outside of their disease state. They are more than just people with disease. The goal is to focus on health, rather than disease management.

PCC considers the person's values, desires, family, social context, and needs in the design or delivery of care. Clinicians and other healthcare workers are also regarded as people and their own physical and mental well-being is paramount to enable them to deliver PCC.

Ideally, care is provided when, how, and in the way it is wanted, as opposed to being provided in the most convenient way for the professionals—or the in most financially efficient way for the provider organizations. PCC commences with the commissioning and design of services, and then in the way we partner with people in clinical interactions.

In Fig. 5.1, the different stages are indicated for commissioning and clinical interactions. Most organizations and clinicians start the PCC journey at the lower rung of the co-production ladder. The change in the way we deliver care has become more important as healthcare has become more complex. Integration of care is essential for people with complex conditions.

The COVID-19 pandemic has demonstrated the benefits of integrated care which is co-produced with people and the communities. The International Foundation for Integrated Care has identified nine key actions that are important to develop PCC (Box 5.2) (Lewis and Ehrenberg, 2020).

A leader for PCC will focus on each of these steps to facilitate delivery of PCC. The interventions described in this chapter will assist clinicians on this journey.

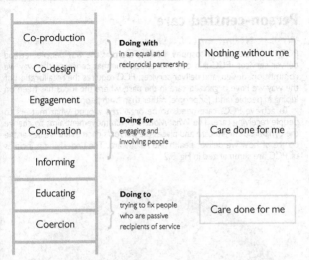

Fig. 5.1 Co-production ladder.

Adapted with permission from Think Local Act Personal (https://www.thinklocalactpersonal.org.uk/co-production-in-commissioning-tool/co-production/In-more-detail/what-makes-co-production-different/).

Box 5.2 Interventions to realign healthcare

- Developing solutions in and for the local context.
- Prioritizing health as opposed to disease.
- People being regarded as partners in their health rather than patients with a disease.
- Building resilient communities.
- Offering digital solutions to assist in the implementation of integrated PCC.
- Educating and transforming the workforce to deliver integrated care.
- Realignment of payment systems to facilitate integrated PCC.
- Introducing transparency in all that we do so that people know what is being planned at every stage, either in commissioning or planning, as well as in clinical management.
- Leadership and governance which is focused on PCC.

From Lewis and Ehrenberg (2020).

Signposting

Think Local Act Personal. *Coproduction.* [online] Available at: https://www.thinklocalactpersonal.org.uk/co-production-in-commissioning-tool/co-production/In-more-detail/what-makes-co-production-different/ (accessed 3/10/2021).

Reference

Lewis, L. and Ehrenberg, N. (2020). *Realising the True Value of Integrated Care.* [online] International Foundation for Integrated Care. Available at: https://integratedcarefoundation.org/publications/realising-the-true-value-of-integrated-care-beyond-covid-19-2#report (accessed 3/10/2021).

Person-centred care

What is person-centred care?

PCC is a healthcare philosophy, which underpins the way people act and deliver services. PCC is a complex endeavour that concerns the way we commission, design, and deliver services. PCC requires the recalibration of the way we have organized care in the past, where the focus has been on 'doing to people' and 'for people' rather than 'with people'.

To achieve PCC, care needs to be organized around what matters to people receiving care. The *What Matters to You* movement aims to change the dynamic of healthcare and places the person's choices and values at the centre of how we deliver health and healthcare. The underlying principles of PCC are summarized in Fig. 5.2.

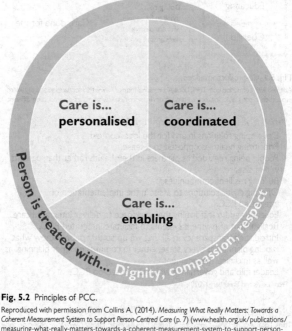

Fig. 5.2 Principles of PCC.

Reproduced with permission from Collins A. (2014). *Measuring What Really Matters: Towards a Coherent Measurement System to Support Person-Centred Care* (p. 7) (www.health.org.uk/publications/measuring-what-really-matters-towards-a-coherent-measurement-system-to-support-person-centred-care).

- *Personalized, safe, quality care* is care that considers the desires and values of the person receiving care even if it is standardized.
- *Coordinated and integrated care* implies that the person receiving the care is in the centre of all planning and delivery and the care is integrated, rather than delivered in silos.

- *Enabling and empowering care* implies that people receiving care are equal partners in the care process and have a say in how and when the care is delivered.

These principles are underpinned by the values of respect, kindness, and compassion, which are often lacking in the technological care processes. Increased health literacy has resulted in a greater focus on the needs of patients as people rather than as individuals with a disease. Healthcare has not always been designed to deliver these principles in that it is organized around the needs of the healthcare system rather than those receiving care.

The chronic care model was developed to assist in the integration of care from both design and delivery perspectives so that productive partnerships and interactions could take place between activated people as patients and their families and activated clinical care teams, supported by the wider system of health, as well as by the community.

The key components for successful management of chronic care are:
- effective community resources and policies:
  - systems and processes to support self-management
- a focused and responsive health system organization:
  - how the system is designed
  - the support provided
  - information technology to facilitate interactions and knowledge sharing
- productive interactions between providers and patients.

This approach can be a foundation for the development of care that places the patient as an equal partner in the development of good outcomes.

Signposting

Kaiser Permanente Washington Health Research Institute. *Chronic Care Model Online Resources*. [online] Available at: http://www.improvingchroniccare.org (accessed 3/10/2021).
The Health Foundation (n.d.). *Person-Centred Care*. Available at: https://www.health.org.uk/topics/person-centred-care (accessed 3/10/2021).
What Matters to You. [online] Available at: https://wmty.world (accessed 3/10/2021).

Further reading

Coleman, K., Austin, B.T., Brach, C., et al. (2009). Evidence on the chronic care model in the new millennium. *Health Affairs*, 28(1), 75–85. doi:10.1377/hlthaff.28.1.75
Collins, A. (2014). *Measuring What Really Matters – A Thought Paper*. London: The Health Foundation. Available at: https://www.health.org.uk/sites/default/files/MeasuringWhatReallyMatters.pdf (accessed 3/10/2021).

Patient experience

What is patient experience?

The implementation of the PCC principles is reflected in the experience that people have of care. Patient experience is defined by The Beryl Institute as 'the sum of all interactions, shaped by an organization's culture, that influence patient perceptions across the continuum of care'. The experience covers all the domains of quality. This differs from patient satisfaction which is about whether expectations have been met. One can have a high satisfaction level even if one has a poor experience and vice versa.

Why is patient experience important?

With the success of modern medical interventions, people are living longer, though with more comorbidities. This has resulted in the need to develop services that are inclusive and integrated. There is evidence that specific person-centred interventions improve quality of care. Good patient experience is correlated with improved patient safety and patient-reported outcomes, although further research is required to support early reports that the person-centred approach as a whole improves outcomes.

What is the theory?

Improving patients' experiences takes time as work systems and processes may need to be redesigned in order to meet the requirements of the underlying PCC principles. This redesign will require a change in the way leaders, managers, and clinicians work, which includes ensuring the following:

- Commissioning and provisioning focus on people rather than diseases.
- Successful strategies prioritize quality and patient safety over a long period and sustain investment in infrastructure and management processes to facilitate and promote PCC.
- Leaders embed the systems and processes required in the organization's culture and way of working to deliver PCC.
- Care delivery is responsive to a person's physical, social, emotional, and cultural needs.
- Staff interactions with persons receiving care are informative, empathetic, and empowering.
- The values and preferences of the person receiving care are elicited and acted upon.
- Reliable health information is readily available.

How does this work in clinical practice?

The principles of PCC include:
- getting to know the patient as a person, recognizing their individuality
- assessing needs holistically, considering family and social circumstances
- recognizing and acknowledging the person's expertise in their own health and care
- sharing power and responsibility based on respect for and promotion of their autonomy
- if possible, allowing people to decide how their care is delivered, with innovations such as people-held budgets to purchase care—by offering

people personal budgets from which they can purchase their own care (e.g. home help)
- making services accessible, flexible, and easy to navigate
- coordinating services into an integrated care pathway
- making the physical, cultural, and psychosocial care environment one that fosters PCC, including having supportive staff with good communication and engagement skills.

As well as an overarching concept that can be internalized by staff, patients and the public, PCC incorporates:
- patient satisfaction and experience
- patient engagement and activation, that is, people are empowered to self-manage and not be dependent on providers of care
- staff kindness, empathy, compassion, and respect for the dignity of the person
- specific staff behaviours such as person-centred communication, facilitating self-management, and shared decision-making
- delivering PCC in turn may have a benefit on the staff's morale and their own mental well-being. Small acts of kindness have been shown to decrease burnout.

Signposting

Mangomoments (n.d.). *Small Acts of Kindness*. [online] Available at: https://mangomoment.org/english-2/ (accessed 3/10/2021).
NHS England (n.d.). *Developing Patient-Centred Care*. [online] Available at: https://www.england.nhs.uk/integrated-care-pioneers/resources/patient-care/ (accessed 3/10/2021).
Planetree International. [online] Available at: https://www.planetree.org/ (accessed 3/10/2021).
The Beryl Institute. [online] Available at: https://www.theberylinstitute.org/ (accessed 3/10/2021).
The King's Fund (2012). *From Vision to Action: Making Patient-Centred Care a Reality*. London: The King's Fund. Available at: https://www.kingsfund.org.uk/sites/default/files/field/field_publication_file/Richmond-group-from-vision-to-action-april-2012-1.pdf (accessed 3/10/2021).

Further reading

Bombard, Y., Baker, G.R., Orlando, E., et al. (2018). Engaging patients to improve quality of care: a systematic review. *Implementation Science*, 13(1). doi:10.1186/s13012-018-0784-z
Merlino, J. (2015). *Service Fanatics: How to Build Superior Patient Experience the Cleveland Clinic Way*. New York: McGraw-Hill Education.

People leading for person-centred care

What is person-centred leadership?

People leading for PCC are flipping the power dynamics and enabling patients as people to lead and manage health and social care services, so as to ensure the delivery of PCC. PCC leadership has been stimulated by healthcare leaders' own experience as patients.

Example of such leadership is the '*Hello my Name is …*' campaign which aims to change the culture and to ensure that all healthcare workers introduce themselves to the patient as a person from the outset to demonstrate empathy, courtesy, compassion, and confidence. Another example is the *What Matters to You* movement which aims to place the person in charge of how and what care is delivered.

Why is it important?

PCC leadership is essential, as the people who know most about healthcare are those receiving the care. It is liked by people as patients and by patient groups, and it is widely promoted by healthcare academics and interest groups. However, the impact or effectiveness is uncertain, as it is unclear as to what really is good person-centred leadership. It requires power sharing by the healthcare hierarchy.

What is the theory?

Patient leaders can contribute to person (patient)-centred leadership. They can face externally, as a community channel, or internally, as a 'critical friend'. Organizations can include person (patient)-centred leaders as board members, as experts by experience, health champions, and peer supporters.

Person (patient)-centred leaders can hold organizations to account, support patients and families, help with understanding patient experience, and improve collaboration. Effective patient leaders have the capacity for 'self-leadership', can focus on solutions, and are willing to value and work with others. They need planning and project management skills.

Patient 'engagement' is often seen by people as an alternative to change, not as part of a change, therefore making the process tokenistic and bureaucratic. The person (patient)-centred leader must shift from the dominant construct of healthcare of the '*child–parent*' dynamic to one of '*equal adults*'. This implies a shift from seeing care as an act from the professional to the patient, to being an act negotiated with the patient as a person or citizen, that is, going up the rungs of the co-production ladder in Fig. 5.1 (see p. 123).

How does this work in practice?

Specific techniques that can help to facilitate PCC leadership include:
- communicating the vision for PCC in the organization at induction
- making PCC a core value, to be assessed at appraisal
- providing meaningful feedback to staff on how they are interacting with people
- rewarding staff members who are successful in providing PCC.

The main resistance to person (patient)-centred leaders may come from health professionals, because of:

- a lack of awareness, knowledge, skills and incentives
- a view that it takes time and resources to be person-centred
- an avoidance of patients' emotional needs
- cultural issues, such as the fear of loss of face, power, income, or an unwillingness to experiment.

The main enablers of PCC are:

- demonstrable leadership from healthcare leaders
- an organizational and team culture that values partnership with people receiving care
- a desire to gain feedback on patient experience, which person-centred leaders are well-placed to provide.

For some tips for success, see Box 5.3.

Box 5.3 Tips for success

- Do not be put off by overwrought terminology or complex literature.
- Be open to the comments, insights, and opinions of patients.
- Include people when making clinical and managerial decisions.

Signposting

Hello my name is ... [online]. Available at: https://www.hellomynameis.org.uk (accessed 3/10/2021).

NHS England (n.d.). *Peer Support*. [online] Available at: https://www.england.nhs.uk/ltphimenu/personalised-care/supported-self-management-peer-support/ (accessed 3/10/2021).

Further reading

Bisognano, M. and Schummers, D. (2014). Flipping healthcare: an essay by Maureen Bisognano and Dan Schummers. *BMJ*, 349(3), g5852–g5852. doi:10.1136/bmj.g5852

de Zulueta, P. (2015). Developing compassionate leadership in health care: an integrative review. *Journal of Healthcare Leadership*, 8, 1–10. doi:10.2147/jhl.s93724

Moore, L., Britten, N., Lydahl, D., et al. (2016). Barriers and facilitators to the implementation of person-centred care in different healthcare contexts. *Scandinavian Journal of Caring Sciences*, 31(4), 662–673. doi:10.1111/scs.12376

O'Hara, J.K., Reynolds, C., Moore, S., et al. (2018). What can patients tell us about the quality and safety of hospital care? Findings from a UK multicentre survey study. *BMJ Quality & Safety*, 27(9), 673–682. doi:10.1136/bmjqs-2017-006974

The King's Fund. (2013). *Patient-Centred Leadership: Rediscovering our Purpose*. London: The King's Fund. Available at: https://www.kingsfund.org.uk/publications/patient-centred-leadership (accessed 3/10/2021).

Vennedey, V., Hower, K.I., Hillen, H., et al. (2020). Patients' perspectives of facilitators and barriers to patient-centred care: insights from qualitative patient interviews. *BMJ Open*, 10(5), e033449. doi:10.1136/bmjopen-2019-033449

Experience-based co-design

What is experience-based co-design?

Experience-based co-design (EBCD) is an approach to redesigning aspects of healthcare services, based on the experience of service users. It focuses on improving the experience of patients and staff in that service, rather than on service improvement more generally.

Why is it important?

It is one of the methods that can lead to the delivery of PCC and thereby better healthcare outcomes.

What is the theory?

Involving patients and carers in the process of altering services, based on experience data leads to improved experience. See Box 5.4.

Box 5.4 EBCD steps

EBCD has five steps:
- Planning.
- Engaging staff and service users to gather experience data.
- Diagnosing the problems with group reflections by staff and service users.
- Prioritizing issues to be addressed in the redesign.
- Co-designing solutions and implementation.

Challenges to EBCD include:
- staff perceiving EBCD activities as an additional burden to their routine work
- lack of additional resources to support the process
- no accountability for implementation of the new design
- high patient throughput, so that co-design is difficult to achieve
- difficulty in engaging service users who may be transient.

Benefits of EBCD include:
- staff, patients, and carers who participate in EBCD activities gain a better understanding of each other's perspectives on a service
- co-designed service improvements are particularly appreciated by service users, because of their direct relevance to their concerns (e.g. privacy, respect, communication, information-sharing between staff)
- the process of EBCD can be accelerated by using videos of service users reporting experience data and sharing the data with many teams offering that kind of service.

How does this work in practice?

EBCD is a partnership between the people receiving care and those planning and delivering care. Narratives and feedback are important, but in EBCD one is looking for the lived experience of the process, and then a re-design of the experience, not only the process that delivers the experience. This includes the subjective experience of people in the process, rather than only objective quantitative measurement.

Signposting

Point of Care Foundation (n.d.). *EBCD: Experience Based Co-Design Toolkit.* [online] Available at: https://www.pointofcarefoundation.org.uk/resource/experience-based-co-design-ebcd-tool kit/ (accessed 3/10/2021).

Further reading

Bate, P. and Robert, G. (2006). Experience-based design: from redesigning the system around the patient to co-designing services with the patient. *Quality and Safety in Health Care,* 15(5), 307–310. doi:10.1136/qshc.2005.016527

Fucile, B., Bridge, E., Duliban, C., et al. (2017). Experience-based co-design: a method for patient and family engagement in system-level quality improvement. *Patient Experience Journal,* 4(2), 53–60. doi:10.35680/2372-0247.1209

Co-production

Co-production is key for improving the quality of healthcare services. It is now recognized that to improve quality, it is important to understand that 'healthcare' is not just 'a product' that is supplied to a patient (which puts the focus on processes, actions, and outputs). Rather, it is a co-produced interaction, considering patient preferences, relationships, and other outcomes that are less easy to measure.

What is the theory?

The theory of co-produced services arose from the economic and business industry in the late 1960s, when it was recognized that the new service economy was different to the old industrial economy. A service involved a different relationship between the producer and consumer.

The idea of co-production has been explored in a variety of public services. It was observed that the public co-produced services by 'locking doors, installing security systems and fire alarms, reporting suspicious activity, sorting garbage and hauling it to the curb and participating in parent–teacher associations' (Batalden et al., 2015).

The co-production of public good was seen to have implications for defining the roles and responsibilities of the public in the service delivery. Customers became known as 'prosumers', able to link production and consumption in a way that maximized their own convenience (e.g. home pregnancy kits, self-service check-outs).

Public bodies and governments have been keen to facilitate improved partnerships between professionals and customers in the co-production of public services. This is a coming together to design and improve services by building on the expertise of the consumer, with resultant increased choice, responsiveness, and reduction of waste and cost.

How does this work in practice?

Co-production involves people who use services, with carers being valued and having an equal, more meaningful, and powerful role in those services (Box 5.5). They are seen as assets with unique knowledge and expertise.

Box 5.5 Example of DIMPLE co-production

An example of co-production of a health service is the Diabetes Improvement through Mentoring and Peer-led Education Project (DIMPLE) in West London. This trained service users and local volunteers, particularly in communities that tended to avoid traditional NHS services, to be diabetes champions, who could educate others about diabetes, and to be peer educators, who could do the same for fellow patients and to act as peer mentors to those undergoing treatment for diabetes.

An evaluation after 18 months showed that 5000 people had been educated. Knowledge, community involvement, support, and professional skills had increased. Patients reported satisfaction with the peer educators and peer mentors and there was anecdotal evidence of mentors helping patients to improve outcomes.

(More information is available at: https://hammersmithandfulhamd iabetes.files.wordpress.com/2013/11/impact-evaluation-of-the-diabe tes-champions-project-mph-dissertation-james-redmore-00718273.pdf)

Power and resources must be transferred from managers to service users or deployed in coordination with them to facilitate the co-production process. Boundaries become blurred with the co-production of services, as the wider network and community become involved.

A necessary corollary of this is that frontline staff also have more involvement in decisions about service delivery. Meaningful interactions between all stakeholders are required to achieve desired outcomes.

Successful co-production requires those who contribute to the service, whether staff or service users, receive something in exchange, such as benefits in kind. Organizations will typically need to alter aspects of their structure, culture, practice, and review arrangements, to engage successfully in co-production. For example, review arrangements will move from the 'you said, we did' model of feedback, to a 'we said, we did' model.

Co-production of health can take place at a clinical level, and involves co-production at every level:

• Assessment of the problem together.
• Deciding on what is required to happen together.
• Designing the plan of action together.
• Delivering care in an equal partnership.

This is the 'Quality 3.0' (see Chapter 3) approach to production of health, rather than the management of disease.

For some tips for success, see Box 5.6.

Box 5.6 Tips for success

• Do not try to get a co-production project off the ground yourself as an organization—seek the advice of organizations like the Coalition for Collaborative Care and the Social Care Institute of Excellence that have programmes for assisting organizations to develop co-production.
• Include service users and carers in the design of the co-production programme.

Signposting

ICoHN International Coproduction Health Network. Available at https://icohn.org/. accessed 9/09/2022

NHS England (2015). *Improving Experience of Care through people who use services.* London: NHS England. Available at: https://www.england.nhs.uk/wp-content/uploads/2013/08/imp-exp-care.pdf (accessed 3/10/2021).

Realpe, A. and Wallace, L.M. (2010). *What is Coproduction?* London: Health Foundation. Available at: https://qi.elft.nhs.uk/wp-content/uploads/2017/01/what_is_co-production.pdf (accessed 3/10/2021).

Further reading

Batalden, M., Batalden, P., Margolis, P., et al. (2015). Coproduction of healthcare service. *BMJ Quality & Safety,* 25(7), 509–517. doi:10.1136/bmjqs-2015-004315

Batalden, P. (2018). Getting more health from healthcare: quality improvement must acknowledge patient coproduction—an essay by Paul Batalden. *BMJ,* 362, k3617. doi:10.1136/bmj.k3617

Batalden, P., Nelson, E., Foster, T. (Editors, 2021) Supplement on coproduction. International Journal for Quality in Health Care, 33 (Supplement_2). Available at: https://academic.oup.com/intqhc/issue/33/Supplement_2. accessed 9/09/2022

Elwyn, G., Nelson, E., Hager, A., et al. (2020). Coproduction: when users define quality. *BMJ Quality & Safety,* 29, 711–716. doi:10.1136/bmjqs-2019-009830

Shared decision-making

What is shared decision-making?

Whereas co-design and co-production focus on a service, shared-decision-making is about the involvement of individual patients in delivering their own personal healthcare.

Why is it important?

Reviews of shared decision-making techniques have found that patients become better informed, take a more active part in making decisions, adhere better to the agreed treatment plan, and often make more conservative decisions (i.e. waiting or avoiding interventions) that can reduce healthcare costs.

What is the theory?

Shared decision-making involves clinicians working together with patients to make joint treatment decisions that consider the relevant evidence base, clinical judgement, and the patient's informed preferences. It aims to provide care that really matters to people.

Shared decision-making has several steps that need to be taken before a decision is made:

- The patient is made aware of the process—*deliberation* of the process.
- *Choices* are then discussed to set the scene for the next phase.
- *Options* of treatment are provided with harms and benefits of each. It requires clinicians to give patients evidence-based information regarding options for tests, treatments, management, and support; the alternatives; the likely consequences of each option; and the degree of uncertainty involved. Decision-support counselling should be available to the patient if the decision involved is a weighty one, as well as tools such as brief decision aids and option grids, if helpful.
- *Decisions* are then made as to how to proceed, and a management plan is agreed.
- Implementing shared decision-making depends crucially on the engagement of senior clinicians, as well as other healthcare leaders. This requires the sharing of evidence on the benefits of shared decision-making, and training staff at all levels in shared decision-making techniques.
- Self-management is a related concept that aims to help people develop the knowledge, skills, and confidence to manage their own health and/ or to recover from an episode of ill health.
- Self-management includes peer support, group education programmes (generic or condition specific; or co-led, including mental health recovery programmes), rehabilitation strategies, motivational interviewing, health coaching, and behaviour change or lifestyle counselling.

How does this work in practice?

Shared decision-making is a complex change in the way clinicians work, so therefore needs active support from clinical leaders (Box 5.7).

The NHS shared decision-making framework indicates the processes needed, from preparing and educating the people receiving care; training, sensitizing, and supporting clinical teams; redesigning pathways and clinical practices; and providing leadership to facilitate the change in practice (Fig. 5.3).

Box 5.7 Example of shared decision-making

An example of shared decision-making is the Health Foundation's Making Good Decisions in Collaboration (MAGIC) programme, which trained staff in primary and secondary care settings in Cardiff and Newcastle in shared decision-making and found that over a relatively short period of time, patients became more confident in managing aspects of their own care.

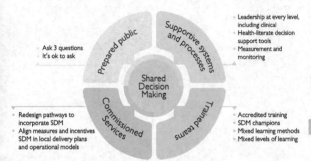

Fig. 5.3 Shared decision-making (SDM) framework (NHS England).
Reproduced with permission from NHS England, under Open Government Licence. https://www.england.nhs.uk/wp-content/uploads/2019/01/shared-decision-making-summary-guide-v1.pdf

Signposting

National Institute for Health and Care Excellence (2021). *Shared Decision Making*. London: National Institute for Health and Care Excellence. Available at: https://www.nice.org.uk/guidance/ng197 (accessed 3/10/2021).

NHS England and NHS Improvement (2019). *Shared Decision Making: Summary Guide*. [online] Available at: https://www.england.nhs.uk/wp-content/uploads/2019/01/shared-decision-making-summary-guide-v1.pdf (accessed 3/10/2021).

The Health Foundation (n.d.). *MAGIC: Shared Decision Making*. [online] Available at: https://www.health.org.uk/funding-and-partnerships/programme/magic-shared-decision-making (accessed 3/10/2021).

Further reading

Ahmad, N., Ellins, J., Krelle, H., et al. (2014). *Person-Centred Care: From Ideas to Action*. London: The Health Foundation. Available at: https://www.health.org.uk/publications/person-centred-care-from-ideas-to-action (accessed 3/10/2021).

Barry, M.J. and Edgman-Levitan, S. (2012). Shared decision making—the pinnacle of patient-centered care. *New England Journal of Medicine*, 366(9), 780–781. doi:10.1056/nejmp1109283

Bomhof-Roordink, H., Gärtner, F.R., Stiggelbout, A.M., et al. (2019). Key components of shared decision making models: a systematic review. *BMJ Open*, 9(12), e031763. doi:10.1136/bmjopen-2019-031763

Coulter, A. and Collins, A. (2011). *Making Shared Decision-Making a Reality: No Decision About Me, Without Me.* London: The King's Fund. Available at: https://www.kingsfund.org.uk/sites/default/files/Making-shared-decision-making-a-reality-paper-Angela-Coulter-Alf-Collins-July-2011_0.pdf (accessed 3/10/2021).

Elwyn, G., Frosch, D., Thomson, R., et al. (2012). Shared decision making: a model for clinical practice. *Journal of General Internal Medicine*, 27(10), 1361–1367. doi:10.1007/s11606-012-2077-6

Stiggelbout, A.M., Van der Weijden, T., De Wit, M.P.T., et al. (2012). Shared decision making: really putting patients at the centre of healthcare. *BMJ*, 344, e256–e256. doi:10.1136/bmj.e256

Technology and digital health

Why is it important?

Technological innovations, such as smartphones and smart watches, have radically altered the ways individuals communicate, share information, and manage aspects of their lives. They have a similar transformative impact on the delivery of healthcare.

The COVID-19 pandemic has demonstrated the value of digital solutions to ensure healthcare is not disruptive—telemedicine, virtual consultation, and video conferencing became the norm. Virtual hospitals have been developed, where people can have vital signs monitored and some investigations, such as electrocardiograms, done remotely.

What is the theory?

Various technologies improve access to, increase the efficiency of, and improve the outcomes of healthcare delivery in various ways:

- Technologies such as regenerative medicine and minimally invasive surgery are perhaps the most familiar and involve new or improved medical interventions.
- Diagnostic technologies, such as nanoscale sensors and point-of-care diagnostics, increase the range, speed, convenience, and accuracy of testing for many different disorders.
- Enabling technologies mitigate the impact of disease and disability, for example, wearable health monitors and assistive technologies, such as speech generators, panic alarms, and mobility devices.
- Preventative technologies reduce the incidence of disease, through the modification of genetic code, or changing lifestyles, using education or game-playing.
- Organizational technologies improve the efficiency and effectiveness of healthcare provision. This is achieved using increasingly interoperable information systems, as well as the analysis and interpretation of 'big data' allowing providers to be compared and outcomes to be assessed on a large scale. This group of technologies is likely to be the most disruptive to healthcare providers.

How does this work in practice?

The following new technologies have been introduced to healthcare:

- RIBA, a robot that can lift patients from a bed or wheelchair and transport them—freeing nurses from the risk of injury through lifting.
- The Nano-retina NR600 replaces the functionality of damaged retinal cells, combining an implant with wireless glasses.
- Smartphone apps to monitor asthma symptoms, moods that could develop into psychosis, and many other symptoms.
- Techniques for reactivating the genes that allow for the regrowth of lost or damaged teeth.
- Computerized avatars that can assist in psychotherapy.
- Electronic underwear that can prevent bedsores.
- CRIS and other software to analyse anonymized healthcare databases for research and other purposes.

See Box 5.8.

Box 5.8 Tips for implementing digital solutions

For sustainable implementation of digital solutions we need:

- to re-educate the workforce to enable them to use the new technologies
- to educate the public on the use and safety of the technologies
- to ensure that the social determinants of access to the technologies and to broadband are addressed
- the co-production of solutions for the use of AI and genomic technologies to be the foundation of the introduction of these innovations
- safety, quality, and person centredness to be at the centre of all that is implemented.

Signposting

NHS Digital. [online] Available at: https://digital.nhs.uk (accessed 3/10/2021).

Further reading

Greenhalgh, T., Koh, G.C.H., and Car, J. (2020). Covid-19: a remote assessment in primary care. *BMJ*, 368, m1182. doi:10.1136/bmj.m1182

Greenhalgh, T., Rosen, R., Shaw, S.E., et al. (2021). Planning and evaluating remote consultation services: a new conceptual framework incorporating complexity and practical ethics. *Frontiers in Digital Health*, 3, 726095. doi:10.3389/fdgth.2021.726095

Greenhalgh, T., Vijayaraghavan, S., Wherton, J., et al. (2016). Virtual online consultations: advantages and limitations (VOCAL) study. *BMJ Open*, 6(1), e009388. http://dx.doi.org/10.1136/bmjopen-2015-009388

Hollander, J.E. and Carr, B.G. (2020). Virtually perfect? Telemedicine for Covid-19. *New England Journal of Medicine*, 382(18), 1679–1681. doi:10.1056/nejmp2003539

Topol E. (2019). *Preparing the Healthcare Workforce to Deliver the Digital Future* ('The Topol Review'). London: HEE. Available at: https://topol.hee.nhs.uk/the-topol-review/ (accessed 3/10/2021).

Measuring person-centred care

Why is it important?

PCC is complex to implement, so therefore needs to be measured to ensure that implementation has been successful. A defined measurement plan can assist organizations and clinicians in the implementation of PCC.

What is the theory?

Measures of PCC are varied and depend on what component one is measuring. Ideally, clinical measures should start with the promotion of health, as well as the encounter with the health service. Measures should measure what matters to people and not only those that matter to the health service. Measures must cover all the domains of quality.

Measures should:

- be capable of assessing experience over the whole pathway of care, considering continuity and coordination, and including transactional elements (e.g. dispensing a prescription) and relational elements (e.g. compassionate communication)
- facilitate assessment against predefined standards. Existing information sources, such as complaints data, should be incorporated; the data currently collected are often poorly interpreted and understood by services and managers
- improve accountability, transparency, and quality. It should align with clinical outcomes (e.g. PROMs), be evidence based, be simple, and be embedded in quality standards (e.g. the ongoing work of the National Institute for Health and Care Excellence (NICE)).

Measures can be at a macro, meso, and micro system level. Some examples are provided in Table 5.1.

Table 5.1 Measurement levels in PCC

Macro system	Degree of co-design and co-production of services Input of PCC leaders in the healthcare decision bodies
Meso and micro system	Measures can include the key principles of PCC: • Compassion, dignity, and respect • Care coordination and integrated care • Empowerment and self-management
Clinical encounter	Patient experience of the clinical consultations and the journey through the system Patient satisfaction with the clinical consultations Patient-reported outcomes Patient-reported experience

Data can be obtained through comment cards, survey questionnaires, in-depth interviews, online ratings focus groups, and personal stories and narratives. These can vary in depth from SMS questions to a more formal questionnaire online, on tablets, or on paper. Validated measures are available to measure individualized care, processes of care, and PCC, with its components.

Complaints and compliments can be a rich source of information. Some websites can offer a site for feedback from patients, though will need moderation to ensure that the comments are related to the care received.

Patient-reported outcome and experience measures (PROMs and PREMs)

(See What is an outcome?, p. 100.)

PROMs are a method of collecting information on the effectiveness of care, as perceived by the patients themselves. PROMs are either generic or disease specific and a combined approach is frequently used. Examples include symptom reduction scales, functional improvement scales, quality of life scales, and disease-specific details. An example of a PROM tool to obtain generic PROM data is the EuroQol five-dimension EQ-5D-5L™.

PREMs are questionnaires measuring the patients' perceptions of their experience while receiving care. They are an indicator of quality of care, rather than a direct measure of it.

PREMs may be functional (in terms of the availability of services), or relational (regarding the relationship with staff). Examples of PREMs include opinions on dignity, cleanliness, trust in the staff, timeliness, etc. Examples of tools to obtain PREMs data are the CARE measure (a relational measure) and the NHS Cancer Patient Experience Survey.

There are many standardized measures used to capture patient-reported outcomes and experiences, applied to a wide variety of settings and at different levels in healthcare services. Patients value the use of PROMs but may not want them to burden the clinical experience or focus on outcomes that are only of interest to clinicians. There is evidence if clinicians use PROMs effectively, clinical outcomes may improve life expectancy in cancer patients. Despite the availability of such measures, attempts to embed them has encountered resistance from clinicians.

The introduction of PROMs and PREMs is a step in the right direction, when considering PCC. However, they do not tell us the full story. One needs to look at outcomes across the entire patient journey to integrate the measurement process. The ICHOM approach can provide a measure of the outcomes at each stage of the patient journey in an integrated manner. They are a patient-centred measurement system, where person-centred activities (or processes) are given their own value. Their relationship with each other and with the person-centred outcome is understood.

Therefore, the focus has shifted to combine the person-centred process with the person-centred outcome. This requires a logical system that always puts the patient at the heart of every step of the process, that is, a patient-centred logic model.

How does this work in practice?

One review found over 150 measures of PCC and patient experience, such as PEECH ('Patient Evaluation of Emotional Care during Hospitalization'). The Individualised Care Scale is an example of a PREM. It tries to measure the degree to which professionals respond to patients' individual needs in hospital. It can be completed by patients, and in another version, by care staff. Studies in the US and Europe have found it to be valid and reliable.

Real-time feedback is used by many organizations to capture patient experience at the point of care delivery. It typically involves a touchscreen with a degree of privacy, on which patients can indicate their satisfaction with various aspects of the care they receive, on simple Likert scales. Results are immediately available to managers, so any comments or complaints can be acted on at once.

For some top tips for measuring PCC, see Box 5.9.

Box 5.9 Top tips for measuring person-centred care

- Define what you are trying to measure, and why, for example:
  - Outcomes.
  - Satisfaction.
  - Experience.
- Decide what kind of data you will collect, for example:
  - Qualitative, providing depth.
  - Quantitative, promoting benchmarking.
- Consider whether every service user should be invited, or a sample. If a sample, how will you ensure the sample is representative?
- Decide when to measure, for example:
  - During episode of care.
  - After episode of care.
  - Both during and after.
- Allocate sufficient time and resources to planning, piloting, implementation, analysis, and dissemination of the results.
- Ensure participants understand why they are being asked for data. Consent is to be obtained for using it, storing it, or sharing it (whichever applies). It is to be compliant with information governance.
- Plan how the information will be used, stored, and anonymized.
- Make sure the system is capable of acting on the results.
- Present the results in several formats to meet the needs of different audiences (e.g. patients, families, staff, managers).

Signposting

International Consortium for Health Outcome Measurement (ICHOM). [online] Available at: https://www.ichom.org (accessed 3/10/2021).

NHS Digital (2021). *Patient Reported Outcomes*. [online] Available at: https://digital.nhs.uk/data-and-information/data-tools-and-services/data-services/patient-reported-outcome-measures-proms (accessed 3/10/2021).

NHS Scotland (2012). *PROMS User Guides*. [online] Available at: http://www.healthcareimprovementscotland.org/our_work/person-centred_care/proms_questionnaire_project/proms_user_guide.aspx (accessed 3/10/2021).

NHS Wales (n.d.). *Patient Reported Outcome Measures*. [online] Available at: https://proms.nhs.wales (accessed 3/10/2021).

Further reading

Basch, E., Deal, A.M., Dueck, A.C., et al. (2017). Overall survival results of a trial assessing patient-reported outcomes for symptom monitoring during routine cancer treatment. *JAMA*, 318(2), 197–198. doi:10.1001/jama.2017.7156

Coulter, A., Locock, L., Ziebland, S., et al. (2014). Collecting data on patient experience is not enough: they must be used to improve care. *BMJ*, 348, g2225–g2225. doi:10.1136/bmj.g2225

de Silva, D. (2013). *Measuring Patient Experience*. London: The Health Foundation. Available at: https://www.health.org.uk/sites/default/files/MeasuringPatientExperience.pdf (accessed 3/10/2021).

de Silva, D. (2014). *Helping Measure Person-Centred Care. A Review of Evidence about Commonly Used Approaches and Tools Used to Help Patient Centred Care.* London: The Health Foundation. Available at: https://www.health.org.uk/publications/helping-measure-person-centred-care (accessed 3/10/2021).

Kingsley, C. and Patel, S. (2017). Patient-reported outcome measures and patient-reported experience measures. *BJA Education*, 17(4), 137–144. doi:10.1093/bjaed/mkw060

Nelson, E.C., Eftimovska, E., Lind, C., et al. (2015). Patient reported outcome measures in practice. *BMJ*, 350, g7818–g7818. doi:10.1136/bmj.g7818

Øvretveit, J., Zubkoff, L., Nelson, E.C., et al. (2017). Using patient-reported outcome measurement to improve patient care. *International Journal for Quality in Health Care*, 29(6), 874–879. doi:10.1093/intqhc/mzx108

van Dael, J., Reader, T.W., Gillespie, A., et al. (2020). Learning from complaints in healthcare: a realist review of academic literature, policy evidence and front-line insights. *BMJ Quality & Safety*, 29(8), 684–695. doi:10.1136/bmjqs-2019-009704

Methods and tools
to implement change

Introduction

An essential part of leadership is the ability to introduce change and then to make the change sustainable. In previous chapters, leadership has focused on what is required to be a leader. In this chapter, the focus will be more on how to implement change.

In clinical care, we work in complex adaptive systems which are systems that require us to constantly adjust to changing demands and challenges. Therefore, we need to be able to lead change and be able to bring the other members of the team along with the change. Several practical tools are discussed, so that leading for change can be practical and easier to do.

Types of change

Transactional change

What is transactional change?

Change can be characterized by its complexity and outcomes. Trying to implement a relatively straightforward change, with mostly predictable outcomes, usually requires transactional change and leadership. This type of change tends to be something that will improve the current situation and ways of working—and the performance of a team or organization.

Why is this important?

Knowing the type of change helps leaders to understand the type of leadership and organizational commitment required. Transactional change requires a leadership style that can maintain performance and make sure that things go smoothly at the current time. Transactional leaders are important to maintain the day-to-day functioning of teams and organizations. However, they can be described as bureaucratic and are usually reactive rather than proactive.

What is the theory?

Transactional leadership is a style that places importance on the 'transaction' or the relationship between a leader and their 'followers'. The leader uses their authority and power to achieve change. A transactional leader does not typically look strategically ahead, so their focus tends to be on planning and execution. This leadership style was first proposed by Weber in 1947, followed by further work by Bass in 1981.

How does it work in practice?

The focus of a transactional leader is typically on the tasks required to achieve the change. Leaders operating in this mode need to define actions, decide and implement policies, and motivate staff to perform the tasks in hand. In these situations, there tends to be only one leader.

For some tips for success, see Box 6.1.

Box 6.1 Tips for success

For this type of change to be successful, it is important to demonstrate the reason for the change and develop capability to undertake the new change.

How do you do this already?

This might be a change to the rota system or a process in everyday workflow, such as ordering a test or investigation.

Transformational change

What is transformational change?

Complex change with unpredictable outcomes, often in a turbulent environment, requires transformational change and leadership. These are changes that completely reshape how things are done, often requiring a radical shift in behaviour and/or culture.

Why is this important?

For transformational change to be successful, new skills, abilities, and ways of thinking are needed. The transformational leadership required encourages innovation and creativity. However, leading transformational change in healthcare can be challenging and this type of change can frequently produce fear, doubt, and insecurity.

What is the theory?

A transformational leader is strategic and looks to the future to take the team or organization to the next level of success, providing a vision for others. Transformational leadership style is characterized by a leader who uses their influence to motivate and enthuse their team, inspiring them to increase their abilities and capabilities. A transformational leader focuses on the enablers for change, including team development, motivation, and collaboration. They use their charisma and enthusiasm to influence others. This leadership style was first described by Burns in 1978.

How does it work in practice?

In transformational change, frequently there is more than one leader in the group. This type of change and leadership promotes innovation and stimulates those involved.

For some tips for success, see Box 6.2.

Box 6.2 Tips for success

When making transformational changes, it is vital that the rationale for the change and the change itself is well communicated, and that those impacted by the change have been involved from an early stage. To undertake this type of change, a leader needs to inspire their people.

How do you do this already?

This type of change might involve trying to introduce a new model of care or completely redesign a clinical pathway, implementing a major new strategy or adopting a radically different technology.

Further reading

Bass, B.M. (1990). From transactional to transformational leadership: learning to share the vision. *Organisational Dynamics*, 18(3), 19–31. doi:10.1016/0090-2616(90)90061-S

Burns, J.M. (1978). *Leadership*. New York: Harper & Row.

Jones, H.B. (2001). Magic, meaning and leadership: Weber's model and the empirical literature. *Human Relations*, 54(6), 753–771. doi:10.1177/0018726701546003

Kotter, J. (2007). Leading change: why transformation efforts fail. *Harvard Business Review*, September. Available at: https://hbr.org/2007/01/leading-change-why-transformation-efforts-fail (accessed 3/10/2021).

Innovation versus change

What is innovation?

Every innovation entails change, but not every change involves innovation. Innovation is about doing things differently or doing different things that may lead to large gains in 'performance'. An innovation may be incremental (building on and improving existing practices), radical (a completely new approach to solving existing problems), or revolutionary (an innovation that creates an entirely new and unexpected market). The different types of innovation can be characterized by their impact on people—'disruptive' or 'non-disruptive'.

While people often think of innovation being technological developments such as medical devices or IT, many innovations are service innovations— the process our patients go through, the way we work, and the way we redesign and develop our health services. Many innovations come from staff working within organizations and close to the frontline (clinicians, managers, and support staff), rather than laboratories or policymakers.

There are many drivers for innovation in healthcare. These include changing demographics, expectations, and advances in knowledge, science, and technology, which create many opportunities for innovation.

Why is this important?

Healthcare is facing unprecedented challenges to improve quality, reduce harm, improve access, increase efficiency, eliminate waste, and lower costs, with increasing expectations and demands. Sometimes the change required might be where there is no established proven way of making the change. Without innovation, many of the advances we have seen in healthcare would not have happened.

What is the theory?

There are different innovation processes, depending on the type of innovation—services, software, drugs, devices, etc. Whatever the type of innovation, there are three common stages:
1. *Invention* (or identification): originating the idea, finding new ways of doing things.
2. *Adoption* (including prototyping and evaluation): testing new ways of doing things and putting the new idea, product, or service into practice, including prototyping, piloting, testing, and evaluating its safety and effectiveness.
3. *Diffusion* (or spread): systematic uptake of the idea, service, or produce into widespread use, or copying across the service.

Healthcare has traditionally been good at invention, but less good at adoption and diffusion.

How does this work in practice?

Searching for and applying innovative approaches to delivering healthcare must become an integral part of the way in which we work. However, in routine clinical practice, habits, patterns, and standardized practices are often safety features that help to achieve high reliability. These patterns need to be acknowledged and purposefully set aside to encourage innovative thinking about how to do things differently and the possibilities and opportunities this might create.

Specific skills are needed to persuade people (staff and patients) to think about innovating something they have become accustomed to and to which they cannot imagine an alternative. People can frequently be resistant to change. Creating innovation is hard work and requires commitment and leadership but is extremely important and rewarding.

For some tips for success, see Box 6.3.

Box 6.3 Tips for success

- Ensure those who are sceptical or posing risks to innovative or creative thinking are included but don't dominate.
- Use creative facilitation techniques and creative thinking sessions (e.g. Edward de Bono's six thinking hats).
- Innovation is as much about applying an idea, service, or product as it is about creating something entirely new, so you don't need to always be the 'inventor'—copying is good!

Signposting

Department of Health (2011). *Innovation Health and Wealth: Accelerating Adoption and Diffusion in the NHS*. London: NHS Institute for Innovation and Improvement/HMSO. Available at: https://web archive.nationalarchives.gov.uk/20130107013731/http://www.dh.gov.uk/en/Publicationsan dstatistics/Publications/PublicationsPolicyAndGuidance/DH_131299 (accessed 3/10/2021).

The de Bono Group (n.d.). *Six Thinking Hats*. [online] Available at: http://www.debonogroup.com/ six_thinking_hats.php (accessed 3/10/2021).

Large-scale change

What is large-scale change?

Large-scale change is change that:

- is widely spread across geographical boundaries, multiple organizations, or multiple distinctive groupings (e.g. doctors, managers, and social care workers)
- is deeply challenging to current mental models and ways of thinking, often because it feels so different from usual
- widely impacts on what people do in their lives or time at work and requires coordinated change in multiple systems.

In order to achieve sustainable large-scale change we must address all three aspects of complex systems: structures, processes, and patterns (SPP).

Why is this important?

Most published literature focuses on changes that are achieved within a 'bounded' system. While there is strong evidence for the methods and approaches for changes in some care delivery (e.g. 'care bundles' for people with diabetes or ventilator care in critical care units), the bigger the change and the more complex the system, the less clear the methods and evidence. However, our efforts to improve patient care are increasingly focusing on those with complex needs, or across a care pathway, often attempting to improve integration of care, and no longer working confined to discrete and well-demarcated areas of health or social care.

What is the theory?

Large-scale change has been studied in the fields of organizational change, engineering, management, leadership, and social science for many years. It has been increasingly focused on healthcare.

There are three dimensions of large-scale change: *pervasiveness, depth, and size* (Fig. 6.1). The further along these three axes, the larger in scale the change.

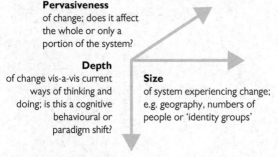

Pervasiveness
of change; does it affect the whole or only a portion of the system?

Depth
of change vis-a-vis current ways of thinking and doing; is this a cognitive behavioural or paradigm shift?

Size
of system experiencing change; e.g. geography, numbers of people or 'identity groups'

Fig. 6.1 Dimensions of large-scale change.

Reproduced from NHS England Sustainable Improvement Team and the Horizons Team (2018). *Leading Large Scale Change: A Practical Guide*, p. 10, under Open Government Licence.

How does this work in practice?

Much of the past change effort in the NHS has focused on the 'S' of SPP—the structures, rather than processes or patterns. To bring about large-scale change in complex systems, it is important to recognize the importance of the last 'P'—patterns in mindsets and behaviours. Often, failure to bring about large-scale change is due to patterns of relationships, decision-making, power, conflict, and learning remaining unchanged and unchallenged. To achieve sustainable large-scale change, all three aspects must be planned for and actively addressed.

Signposting

NHS England (2018). *Leading Large-Scale Change*. London: NHS England. Available at: https://www.england.nhs.uk/wp-content/uploads/2017/09/practical-guide-large-scale-change-april-2018-smll.pdf (accessed 3/10/2021).

Further reading

Bevan, H., Plesk, P., and Winstanley, L. (2011). *Leading Large Scale Change: A Practical Guide*. London: NHS Institute for Innovation and Improvement. Available at: https://www.england.nhs.uk/improvement-hub/wp-content/uploads/sites/44/2011/06/Leading-Large-Scale-Change-Part-1.pdf (accessed 3/10/2021).

Assessing the need for change

There are many tools available to assess the need for change. In this section we will further elaborate on some of those which can be used.

PESTLE analysis

What is a PESTLE analysis?

A PESTLE analysis, sometimes known as a PEST analysis, is a management tool that provides a way of analysing external forces which may be calling for change or that can impact a change project.

Why is a PESTLE analysis important?

It can identify how the principal forces driving change may impact the change process and so be taken into consideration during the change strategy. It provides and analyses different angles and can help teams and organizations prepare for change, by understanding the broader environment, context, and challenges. It can encourage more strategic thinking or highlight opportunities. However, to be effective it needs to incorporate the right amount of data.

What is the theory?

PESTLE is a framework based on an acronym of six elements: P is for Political, E is for Economic, S is for Social, T is for Technological, L is for Legal and E is for Environmental. Sometimes other forces may be added or substituted, such as ethical. See Table 6.1.

Table 6.1 PESTLE analysis—examples of drivers influencing change in healthcare

Driver	Examples in healthcare
Political/policy	Government healthcare policy—choice, competition, healthcare organization
Economic	Cost pressures, funding arrangements, workforce factors
Social	Patient expectations, demographic factors
Technological	New advances in technology or clinical techniques, changes in IT systems
Legal	Clinical safety directives, medical device legislation, litigation, regulation
Environment	Incorporating sustainable practices into the supply chain, use of estates and facilities

How does this work in practice?

A PESTLE analysis should be conducted when developing a new strategy or making a business case for significant change. Once the elements of the PESTLE have been identified, they can be used to build up the external factors for the 'opportunities' and 'threats' in a SWOT analysis (see SWOT analysis, p. 152). For instance, if a hospital is planning to close an outpatient service, this would appear under 'Political' and could be transferred to the SWOT analysis as an opportunity ('O') to save money or may be a threat ('T') to quality of care, such as access.

For some tips for success, see Box 6.4.

Box 6.4 Tips for success

Conducting a PESTLE analysis as a team will help provide a comprehensive analysis by including different perspectives and viewpoints. This may also allow the team to collectively focus on important issues. There are lots of templates available to help conduct a PESTLE analysis.

How do you do this already?

You may implicitly address some of these factors when making changes.

SWOT analysis

What is a SWOT analysis?

A tool used to evaluate strengths and weaknesses from within an organization, and the opportunities and threats from external sources which are driving or may have an impact on a change project.

Why is this important?

A SWOT helps clarify what areas need to change and the capabilities that exist within the organization, to begin to frame the change. A SWOT analysis can help build the case for change. A SWOT analysis can help identify opportunities, manage, and eliminate threats to change.

What is the theory?

A SWOT involves specifying the objective of the change project and identifying the internal and external factors that are favourable and unfavourable to achieving that objective. Strengths (S) and Weaknesses (W) are often internal to the organization, while Opportunities (O) and Threats (T) usually relate to external factors.

How does it work in practice?

A SWOT analysis is important for making a case for change and may be used as part of strategy development or putting forward a business case (Table 6.2). It can be used in conjunction with a PESTLE analysis.

For some tips for success, see Box 6.5.

Table 6.2 Use a SWOT analysis to identify:

	EXTERNAL	
	Opportunities, e.g. collaboration with other teams, organizations	Threats, e.g. financial constraints, other services or organizations, contract impositions
Strengths, e.g. financial position, quality, performance, research, capabilities	How will you maximize these strengths to exploit these opportunities?	How will you maximize these strengths to reduce the impact of these threats?
Weaknesses, e.g. inadequate systems, lack of data, limitations on estates	How will you overcome these weaknesses to exploit these opportunities? Or list opportunities as actions that can be taken to tackle the weaknesses	How will you minimize these weaknesses to stop these threats becoming reality?

(Left side labeled: **INTERNAL**)

Box 6.5 Tips for success

- It is best to conduct a SWOT analysis as a team effort. Avoid downplaying threats or weaknesses, as they will affect the change process at a later stage. The goal is not to neutralize any weakness, but to have it on the radar—and where possible take avoiding action.
- Whether the origin of the change is internal to the organization or external will influence how individuals respond to it. Internal drivers for change may make people feel more in control of events and proactive in exploiting opportunities. External drivers of change (e.g. imposition of a new working contract) may make people less positive and disruptive to the change effort.

Further reading

Kotter, J. and Schlesinger, L. (2008). Choosing strategies for change. *Harvard Business Review*, July–August. Available at: https://hbr.org/2008/07/choosing-strategies-for-change

Process mapping

What is process mapping?

This a technique used in change and improvement. A process map visually represents the steps in a process or pathway. It helps provide a common understanding of the current process and enables identification of opportunities for change and improvement to be made. It provides information on what is done by whom and how things flow. It can help identify issues with flow and waste, as well as provide indicators for gaining further information, such as understanding staff or patient experience at particular points on the pathway.

Why is this important?
Delivery of healthcare is more than the tasks performed by different individuals and parts of the system. Understanding the whole process, rather than individual tasks, is paramount to change and improvement. Creating a process map should be a collective activity undertaken by those who provide and use the pathway. The process map is also an important communication tool for engaging people in the process.

What is the theory?
Process maps are also known as flowcharts, process charts, or workflow diagrams. Process mapping can be used to help identify bottlenecks, repetition, delays, and boundaries. It also helps to identify ownership and responsibilities, and to define measures or metrics. It is common to create two versions—the current state ('As Is'), and the desired future state ('To Be'). There are different types of process mapping. Common types include:
* conventional mapping
* value stream mapping—a LEAN management tool that analyses the steps in relation to value to the customer
* swim lane mapping—separates out the processes according to those responsible for the process.

Key elements in process mapping include activity and decision points. There are standard symbols to use for drawing the process as shown in Fig. 6.2:
* A box shows the activities of the process.
* A diamond represents the stage where a decision is required.
* An oval shows the start of a process and the inputs required. It is used to mark the end of the process with the results or outputs. This will emphasize interdependency.
* Arrows show direction or flow of the process.

How does it work in practice?

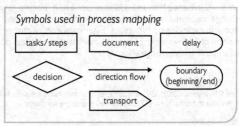

Fig. 6.2 Process mapping symbols.

To develop an accurate representation, those with direct experience of the process need to be involved in mapping. Where this is not possible, the process should be directly observed. People frequently have different views of what is going on in the pathway.

For some tips for success, see Box 6.6.

How do you do this already?

Box 6.6 Tips for success

It is important to define the scope or start and end points to create boundaries. These steps can be followed to create a process map:
- Identify the problem.
- Generate a list of activities involved.
- Determine the sequencing.
- Draw the process map.
- Agree and finalize the process map.

Developing algorithms or clinical guidelines requires an understanding of the process and a process map will differentiate between the work as is and the work as imagined in the guideline.

Signposting

NHS Innovation and Improvement (2021). *Conventional Process Mapping*. London: NHS Innovation and Improvement. Available at: https://www.england.nhs.uk/wp-content/uploads/2021/03/qsir-conventional-process-mapping.pdf (accessed 3/10/2021).

Root cause analysis

What is root cause analysis?

If a system is perfectly designed to achieve the results that are achieved, how do we come up with ideas to change and improve it? While one is working within a well-worn system it can be difficult to think beyond this system. Some simple techniques can help us explore what changes will lead to an improvement. Root cause analysis (RCA) is one method to use to identify issues to be addressed. It must be made part of a larger problem-solving effort for quality improvement.

RCA is a collective term that describes a wide range of techniques that are used to uncover causes of problems. Some approaches are targeted at truly identifying root causes, while some are more general problem-solving techniques. See Box 6.7.

Box 6.7 Root cause analysis

Goals and benefits
- Diagnose the root cause of the problem not just symptoms.
- Understand how to eliminate or mitigate vulnerabilities and learn from root cause.
- Prevent future issues or learn how to replicate good practice.

Key principles
- Focus should be on corrective action rather than the symptoms.
- Be methodical and gather enough information and data to effect change.
- There may be more than one root cause.
- Provide enough information and data to effect change.
- RCA is not about blame: it is how and why, not who.
- Plan to prevent future root causes.
- Buy-in from stakeholders, clients, or patients is essential.

Approaches to root cause analysis

The key to solving a problem is to first understand it. Often, we jump from problem to solution, before really understanding its root cause. What we think is the cause may just be a symptom. A systematic approach to RCA is essential. There are many methodologies, approaches, and technique to help one conduct an RCA. In this section, we will look at two methods in more detail. When carrying out RCA methods and processes, it is important to note:

- while many RCA tools can be used by a single person, the outcome generally is better when a group of people work together to find the problem causes
- those ultimately responsible for removing the identified root cause(s) should be prominent members of the analysis team that sets out to uncover them.

A *typical design of an RCA* in an organization might follow these steps:

1. Form a small team to conduct the RCA.
2. At the analytic phase the emphasis is placed on defining and understanding the problem, brainstorming its possible causes, analysing causes and effects, and devising a solution to the problem.
3. Regular short meetings, at a maximum of 2 hours. As they are meant to be creative in nature, the agenda is quite loose.
4. Roles and tasks assigned to team members.
5. Solution designed.
6. Implementation phase, which depends on what is involved. This may be a very quick or ongoing process, over weeks to months.

There is an array of methods for performing a RCA including but not limited to five whys, fishbone diagrams, failure mode and effects analysis (FMEA), and Pareto diagrams. Here we will focus on two simple common methods—five whys and fishbone diagrams.

Five whys

What is five whys?

This method originated from Toyota's lean manufacturing. It looks to identify the root cause of a problem by asking 'Why?', as many times as needed until the root cause and not just the symptoms, is established (Box 6.8). Depending on the issue, you may need to ask fewer or more questions.

> **Box 6.8 How to run a five whys session**
>
> - Define the issue in plain language. The problem should be a pattern and not just as an isolated event.
> - Choose a person to lead the discussion and assign responsibilities for solutions the group uncovers.
> - Ask 'Why?' until you get to the root cause of the problem.
> - Explore the best way to solve the problem and make the subsequent changes to the system to ensure it doesn't happen again.
> - Communicate changes made.

The five whys serve as a way to avoid assumptions. By finding detailed responses to incremental questions, answers become clearer and more concise each time. Ideally, the last 'Why?' will lead to a process that failed, one which can then be fixed. The five whys is most useful when the problem involves human factors and interactions.

It may not explore all the underlying problems and is probably not suited to large complex problems. In these instances, a cause-and-effect analysis may be more beneficial.

Signposting

NHS England (n.d.). *Using Five Whys to Review a Simple Problem.* [online] Available at: https://www.england.nhs.uk/wp-content/uploads/2022/02/qsir-using-five-whys-to-review-a-simple-problem.pdf (accessed 3/10/2021).

Further reading

Card, A.J. (2016). The problem with '5 Whys'. *BMJ Quality & Safety*, 26(8), 671–677. doi:10.1136/bmjqs-2016-005849

Fishbone diagram

What is the fishbone (cause-and-effect) diagram?

The fishbone diagram, also known as the Ishikawa diagram or cause-and-effect diagram, is a tool which helps to visually display the many potential causes for a specific problem or effect (Fig. 6.3). It is so-called as the diagram looks like a fish skeleton, and it is particularly useful in a group setting and for situations in which little quantitative data are available for analysis. It can generate lots of ideas and expand breadth of thinking as to the problem's root cause. In addition, the exercise usually generates lots of ideas and expands scope of thinking as to the problem's root cause, resulting in a better understanding of the problem, so leading to an effective and durable solution (Box 6.9).

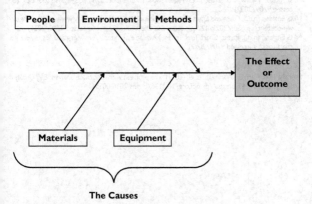

Fig. 6.3 Example of a fishbone diagram.
Reproduced with permission from East London NHS Foundation Trust.

Box 6.9 How to construct a fishbone diagram

1. Start with the problem in the form of a question, such as 'Why is the help desk's abandon rate so high?' Framing it as a 'why' question will help in brainstorming, as each root cause idea should answer the question. The team should agree on the statement of the problem and then place this question in a box at the 'head' of the fishbone.
2. Draw a horizontal line across the page to the left attached to the problem statement. This is the spine.
3. The rest of the bone are lines drawn vertically from the spine and are labelled with different categories. The categories you use are up to you to decide. There are a few standard choices. In a health system they might include the following: people, procedures, environment, equipment, and materials.
4. For each category, generate a list of the causes that contribute to the effect. They may require branch bones to show sub-causes, allowing the true drivers of a problem to be determined.

The fishbone diagram can be combined with five whys methodology to explore the causes identified. For each cause identified, continue to ask, 'Why does that happen?' and attach that information as another bone.

Once you have the fishbone completed, you are well on your way to understanding the root causes of your problem. It would be advisable to have your team prioritize in some manner the key causes identified on the fishbone. If necessary, you may also want to validate these prioritized few causes with a larger audience.

Signposting

Institute for Healthcare Improvement. *Failure Modes and Effects Analysis (FMEA) Tool*. Available at: https://www.ihi.org/resources/Pages/Tools/FailureModesandEffectsAnalysisTool.aspx (accessed 9/09/2022)

NHS England (n.d.). *Cause and Effect (Fishbone)*. [online] Available at: https://www.england.nhs.uk/wp-content/uploads/2021/12/qsir-cause-and-effect-fishbone.pdf (accessed 3/10/2021).

NHS England (n.d.). *Pareto Chart Tool*. [online] Available at: https://www.england.nhs.uk/pareto-chart-tool/ (accessed 9/09/2022)

Further reading

Peerally, M.F., Carr, S., Waring, J., et al. (2017). The problem with root cause analysis. *BMJ Quality & Safety*, 26, 417–422. http://dx.doi.org/10.1136/bmjqs-2016-005511

Assessing variation

What is variation?

Healthcare is complex, with a large amount of variation, namely that there are differing levels of service need, quality, provision, etc. Variation can be seen in a variety of ways, including clinical activity, processes of care, expenditure, outcomes, performance, and access. In some cases, there is good reason for variation, but in other cases this can have a detrimental impact on patient care and available resources.

Why is this important?

The important thing is not to eliminate all variation, but to differentiate between 'bad variation', also known as unwarranted variation, and good variation, known as 'warranted variation' (Table 6.3). Unwarranted variation provides opportunities for improvements, so can lead to greater efficiency, productivity, and improved quality of care.

Table 6.3 Warranted and unwarranted variation

Warranted variation	Unwarranted variation
• Each patient is different and needs to be cared for as an individual with specific symptoms, characteristics, needs, personal circumstances, and values (NHS Constitution)	• Random or occurring by chance
	• Not enough use of high-value or evidenced-based interventions by people from lower socioeconomic backgrounds or 'hard-to-reach' groups
• Variation based on the assessed need of the population served	• Too much use of lower-value interventions—steps that waste NHS resources risk treatment where it isn't essential or of the highest value to the individual
• Innovations in treatments or care need to be tested before they are adopted across all settings.	

What is the theory?

Some variation seen in healthcare can be harmful for patients and families, as well as for healthcare systems. Not all variation that is found in healthcare is 'bad'. Some variation is 'good' and justified. This type of variation is a result of appropriate shared decision-making, patient choice, and PCC. Variation may also occur due to the introduction of innovation. Initially, variation may be seen but decreases as the innovation becomes more widespread.

Causes of variation can largely be characterized by variation in demand and variation in supply (Fig. 6.4).

Variations seen in data can also be due to chance or random occurrences seen in data. 'Common cause variation' is variation that is inherent in a process and occurs frequently and randomly. This is different from 'special cause variation' which is variation that is not usually part of a process but occurs because of specific circumstances.

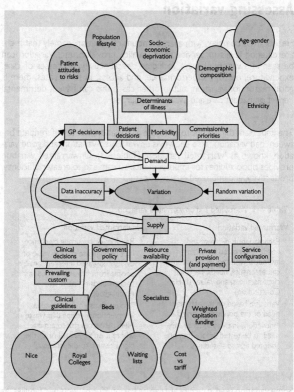

Fig. 6.4 Causes of variation in healthcare systems (based on systems in England).

Reproduced with permission from Appleby, J., et al. (2011). *Variations in Health Care: The Good, the Bad and the Inexplicable*, The Kings Fund, p. 3.

How does it work in practice?

Tackling variation is complex and requires different interventions. These include:

* ensuring data on variation are systematically and routinely collected and published
* supporting clinicians to utilize data to identify variation
* tackling unwarranted variation, including encouraging development and use of protocols and guidelines.

Graphs and statistical techniques can be used to help measure variation. Graphical data enables people to see the impact of decisions on variation. Run charts and SPC charts are used to examine variation to help to assess which type of variation is occurring and whether the changes that are made are having an impact. There are several 'rules' that help you assess whether you have special cause or common cause variation (see Chapter 4).

For some tips for success, see Box 6.10.

Box 6.10 Tips for success

Addressing variation may be unfamiliar to some clinicians and managers. As well as investing efforts in collecting and publishing appropriate data, developing skills to analyse and interpret data is also important.

Run charts are simple to create and should be adequate for most of the measurement display. There may be occasions where you need to use an SPC chart to specifically understand how much variation exists.

How do you do this already?

Reviewing data about performance such as average waiting times for a service over time plotted as a run chart.

Further reading

The King's Fund (2011). *Variations in Healthcare*. London: The Kings Fund. Available at: https://www.kingsfund.org.uk/sites/default/files/field/field_publication_file/Variations-in-health-care-good-bad-inexplicable-report-The-Kings-Fund-April-2011.pdf (accessed 3/10/2021).

Engaging the stakeholders

What is stakeholder mapping?

Stakeholders are the interested and potentially interested parties in a project. These are people who can influence and affect the project as well as those who are influenced and affected by the project. These may be people who are closely or frequently involved in the project or more distant and may not know about the project. At the outset of a change, it is important to map and analyse the stakeholders (Fig. 6.5).

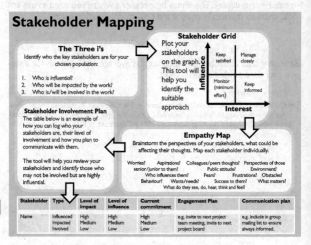

Fig. 6.5 Stakeholder analysis table.
Reproduced with permission from East London NHS Foundation Trust.

Why is this important?

Involving the right people and understanding their perspectives will help to ensure that change is implemented and sustained. Identifying who might be a supporter or a blocker is an important part of this. Stakeholders can be involved in different ways including sponsoring the change project or giving advice and expert input.

What is the theory?

The first stage involves identifying all relevant stakeholders. It is important to think of all the people who might be affected. Once a list of stakeholders has been generated, the second stage is to categorize according to their power, influence, and the extent to which they might be impacted by the change. It is also important to understand the stakeholders and think about the level of desired support and the roles the stakeholders might play, if any.

How does it work in practice?

The 'C' framework can be used to help identify stakeholders. These are as follows:

- *Commissioners:* those who pay for things.
- *Customers:* those who acquire and use the services and products.
- *Collaborators:* those worked with to develop and deliver services or products.
- *Channels:* those who provide the route to the customer.
- *Commentators:* those whose opinions are heard by customers and others.
- *Champions:* those who believe in and will actively promote the project.
- *Competitors:* those working in the same area who offer similar or alternative services.

For some tips for success, see Box 6.11.

Box 6.11 Tips for success

- Gather a diverse group of people to help identify stakeholders and brainstorm a list. A whiteboard or flipchart is a simple way to brainstorm.
- Once they have been identified, they can begin to be aligned to their level of interest and involvement using a simple grid or chart.

Communicating the programme

Once identified, a communication plan is required to run the course of the project so that all stakeholders are kept informed and engaged. This is continually updated, and innovative ways of communication need to be considered such as email, posters, social media, etc. A communication plan needs to be vibrant and in real time.

Signposting

NHS Improvement (2021). *Stakeholder Analysis.* London: NHS Improvement. Available at: https://www.england.nhs.uk/wp-content/uploads/2021/03/qsir-stakeholder-analysis.pdf (accessed 13/1/2021).

Stakeholder analysis

Tool: commitment of continuum analysis

What is commitment of continuum analysis?

A tool that helps provide insight into how much and what sort of influence is needed to move stakeholders towards committing to a change project.

Why is this important?

Understanding the beliefs and needs of the stakeholder aids thinking about ways to frame the need for change and about how to attract supporters. It helps understand and target time and energy at the right stakeholders that must be persuaded to commit to a project. It is often the transition that people resist rather than the change itself, so it is important to realize the different stages people may go through when experiencing a change.

What is the theory?

Not everyone involved in a change project will be fully committed to it. People involved in a change project will position themselves at various points along a continuum in response to proposed action and change. People may range in their responses along a continuum from fully committed to non-compliant (Fig. 6.6). Influencing stakeholders to move along the continuum requires mindset change to help them to come to terms with a change. Some change can happen quickly, but it can take individuals a while to adjust.

Stakeholder	Obstructing	No commitment	Let it happen	Help it happen	Make it happen
A		X			O
B				X —— O	
C			O		X
D	X		O		

X = Current position   O = Where we need them to be for change

Fig. 6.6 Continuum of commitment analysis table.

Reproduced with permission from NHS Improvement (2018). *Leading Large Scale Change: A Practical Guide*. London: NHS Improvement. Available at: https://www.england.nhs.uk/wp-content/uploads/2017/09/practical-guide-large-scale-change-april-2018-smll.pdf

How does it work in practice?

- Identify the key stakeholders using stakeholder mapping.
- Identify their likely response to the change.
- Identify actions that may move each group along the continuum to a more positive mindset, so you know where to focus your drive for commitment.

STAKEHOLDER ANALYSIS **165**

For some tips for success, see Box 6.12.

Box 6.12 Tips for success
- You are more likely to accomplish change if you analyse what level of support you need from each of the participants, and then direct your energy towards achieving it, rather than trying to persuade everybody to commit.
- Wholehearted commitment from everybody is not necessary for change to succeed.

Further reading

Bridges, W. (2017). *Managing Transitions: Making the Most of Change*, 4th ed. London: Nicholas Braealy Publishing.

NHS Improvement (2018). *Leading Large Scale Change: A Practical Guide*. London: NHS Improvement. Available at: https://www.england.nhs.uk/wp-content/uploads/2017/09/practical-guide-large-scale-change-april-2018-smll.pdf (accessed 3/10/2021).

Winning hearts and minds

What is winning hearts and minds?

Winning hearts is about connecting people at an emotional level to the change. Winning minds is about constructing a well-articulated position about the change supported by logic and data.

Why is this important?

Change is about people. It is about doing things differently. In order to persuade people effectively, we need to win both hearts and minds.

What is the theory?

Winning hearts is about connecting with people on a personal level. Metaphors help draw people into a vision and sharing stories and experiences helps to demonstrate that the proposed changes are something that should be supported. Winning minds is about articulating a position and an analysis of the situation to support the change.

How does it work in practice?

Some circumstances may call for one approach over another. For example, prioritizing winning hearts may be preferred when trying to gain support for a new idea, a decision that is already made, or bringing together people who are in conflict. It may be helpful to focus on winning minds when trying to change the direction of something already decided or advocating one choice over another—or asking those with an analytical preference to buy into the change.

For some tips for success, see Box 6.13.

Box 6.13 Tips for success

In most situations, an element of both approaches will be required. However, it is important to pay careful attention to the audience. Giving equal weight to both emotion and logic can be less engaging and influential. Try to identify the strongest position based on the circumstance.

Further reading

Lai, L. (2015). Focus on winning either hearts or minds. *Harvard Business Review*, 20 May. Available at: https://hbr.org/2015/05/focus-on-winning-either-hearts-or-minds (accessed 3/10/2021).

Shaikh, U. and Lachman, P. (2021). Using the Head, Heart, And Hands to Manage Change in Clinical Quality Improvement in the Time of COVID-19. IJQHC Communications. doi:10.1093/ijcoms/lyab012.

Spreading and sustaining change

What is spreading and sustaining change?

Spreading and sustaining change is not easy. Healthcare has a long history of developing innovations, but the spread of these has often been slow. The ability to close the gap between 'best practice' and 'common practice' in part depends on the ability of those leading change to influence and rapidly disseminate innovation and ideas (Horton et al., 2018). Once change or improvement is underway, it can be a challenge to maintain interest and engagement in the project.

Why is this important?

Change frequently requires changes in behaviour and constant effort. Careful planning and building proper foundations mean that implementing and sustaining change can be easier and have a higher chance of success.

What is the theory?

Spread refers to something that is disseminated across an organization or system. It usually involves implementing an intervention or innovation that is proven or based on best practice. *Sustainability* is when new ways of working become the norm and are embedded into everyday practice. The diffusion adoption curve suggests five different categories of adopters to change (Fig. 6.7). These are innovators, early adopters, early majority, late majority, and laggards. They may sit 'within' or 'outside' the community. The adoption of a new idea follows an S-shaped curve when plotted over time.

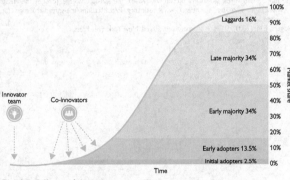

Fig. 6.7 Diffusion of innovation.
Reproduced with permission from, Horton, T., et al. (2018). *The Spread Challenge*, The Health Foundation, p. 37.

How does it work in practice?

Spread and sustainability are complex issues and have been widely studied within and outside healthcare. Rogers (2003) identified six key innovation attributes which have been shown to increase the likelihood of spread:

- *Relative advantage:* the degree to which the change is perceived as being better than the idea it supersedes.

- *Compatibility:* the degree to which the change is perceived as being consistent with the existing values, past experiences, and needs of potential adopters.
- *Trialability:* the degree to which the change can be tested before full adoption.
- *Visibility and observability:* the ability to see the benefits.
- *Timescale:* this includes the timing of introduction, and the time it takes to adopt the change.

For some tips for success, see Box 6.14.

Box 6.14 Tips for success

Talk about progress regularly and tell success stories and stories about learning the change process. People need to see the point of engaging in change and doing things differently. Role modelling is an important aspect of change. It is important to see leaders and senior colleagues embrace change. Systems, processes, and incentives need to be aligned to and support the change in order for it to be widely adopted and sustained.

Signposting

The Health Foundation (2015). *Communications in Health Care Improvement—A Toolkit.* London: The Health Foundation. Available at: https://www.health.org.uk/publications/communications-in-health-care-improvement-a-toolkit (accessed 3/10/2021).

References

Horton, T., Illingworth, J., and Warburton, W. (2018). *The Spread Challenge.* [online] The Health Foundation. Available at: https://www.health.org.uk/publications/the-spread-challenge (accessed 3/10/2021).

Rogers, E.M. (2003). *Diffusion of innovations.* 5th ed. New York: Free Press.

Leadership for clinical education

Introduction

The success of a health system is dependent on the development of a learning environment in which both those receiving care and those delivering care are in a constant learning cycle. Education needs to be continuous with the aim of ensuring the development of shared learning.

Along with the acquisition of the knowledge of medical conditions and the practical tools to deliver treatment, healthcare professionals must acquire the skills of effective systems leadership, management, and interprofessional collaboration to deliver high-quality, safe, and effective care in the twenty-first century. Learning needs to be shared so that all professionals have a common understanding of how the system works, to achieve the desired outcomes.

Clinical education has an important role to enhance the delivery of high-quality, safe PCC by effectively training the healthcare workforce for the future demands of integrated care. All clinicians will be teachers and lifelong learners, as they progress along their careers.

The aim should be to develop a learning system in which all clinicians learn continually from experience, as well as from the didactic approach. The experience of the COVID-19 pandemic emphasized the importance of rapid learning and adaptation of the way systems work. Learning organizations learn every day from every interaction and adapt and improve processes to achieve the desired outcomes.

Further reading

Bohmer, R., Shand, J., Allwood. D., et al. (2020). Learning systems: managing uncertainty in the new normal of Covid-19. *NEJM Catalyst*, 16 July. Available at: https://catalyst.nejm.org/doi/full/10.1056/CAT.20.0318 (accessed 3/10/2021).

Designing and assessing how an education programme works in different contexts

Education programmes range from didactic teaching to experiential learning and then to coaching and mentoring. Healthcare systems are complex, and if we want to continually improve care we need to understand how to learn in different environments. To ensure the programme is appropriate for different contexts, the programme can be assessed using realistic evaluation methodology.

When one designs a learning programme, there are several stages to include to ensure success, as shown in Table 7.1.

Table 7.1 Learning processes and examples

Learning process	Example of learning
Acquisition of knowledge	Reading a text, attending a learning session
Inquiry and investigation	Searching for more information on the internet, reading papers
Discussion	Discussion with peers and colleagues to share learning and to gain further understanding
Practice	Apply the theory on action in the clinical setting, e.g. if one learns about heart sounds, one then examines a patient's heart
Collaboration	Apply the learning within the clinical team, learn together so that there is shared understanding, e.g. inter-professional learning
Produce	Achieve the desired learning and clinical outcomes by putting the theory into practice. This can also be the outcome of the learning

Based on Laurillard (2002).

The success of the programme needs to be assessed and this can be part of programme design and ongoing refinement. Realistic evaluation is a method to achieve ongoing improvements in education.

What is a realist evaluation?

Realist evaluation, developed by Pawson and Tilley (Pawson, 2013; Pawson and Tilley, 1997) is based on the philosophy of realism. The goal of realist evaluation is to understand how education programmes work in different contexts. For example, how does a patient safety programme work in different units of a hospital and within different clinical teams? The aim is to explain 'how', 'why', and for whom, in what circumstances, and to what extent the programme works (Box 7.1).

The approach is based on the following assumptions:
- There are multiple components, both human and material, which make up the learning intervention.
- Interactions between the different components produce the learning outcomes.
- The various interactions do not interact in a linear and deterministic way with each other, that is, a learner may not learn from a lecture and there may be interacting pathways that determine the learning outcome.

Box 7.1 Realistic evaluation

Realist evaluation addresses the following questions:
- What theories of change are embedded in the educational programme?
- What do the stakeholders (i.e., the designers, teachers, and practitioners) think the training achieves, why, and how?
- What data do they collect to evaluate the training and why?
- Are the theories of change substantiated by the collected data and are they supported by relevant research literature?

Why is it important?

Realist evaluation is important because it generates understanding about our educational interventions. This enables causal inferences to be made about how programmes might best be made to work in the future and the connections between the theoretical assumptions and principles which underlie (complex) interventions. This became more important during the COVID-19 pandemic when in-person learning was converted to virtual learning.

What is the theory?

Knowledge acquisition is a complex and dynamic as well as a social and historical product. To evaluate effectiveness of a programme, one must consider the social, political, and cultural context of interventions as well as the theoretical mechanisms that underpin the learning. The purpose of realist evaluation is to test or refine programme theories as well as to see how the programme works in a particular setting. It answers the hypothesis 'if we apply this learning, then an outcome can be expected in this context', and to determine what works, for whom, and under which circumstances in a real-world situation.

A 'CMO' is a hypothesis that the programme works (outcome; O) because of the action of some underlying mechanism (M) which only comes into operation in particular contexts (C) (Box 7.2). These are then used to produce *middle range theories* of what will work and can be tested in different contexts.

They are a generalization of the original theory to determine what type of education intervention will work in different learners in different contexts, and what explains this pattern of learning. Middle range theories are most useful as they are specific enough to test certain proposals yet

Box 7.2 Key components of realistic evaluation

Intervention programmes do not necessarily work for everyone because people and contexts are different. A hypothesis is established regarding the education programme, that is, if we do something, a specific outcome will be achieved. Qualitative and quantitative data are collected and based on these, hypotheses about how *contexts* and *mechanisms* interact to produce *outcomes* (the CMOs of the programme)

$$Contexts + Mechanisms = Outcomes$$

Contexts

Context influences reasoning and generative mechanisms can only work if the circumstances are right. Context may provide alternative explanations of the observed outcomes.

Mechanisms

Mechanisms are the underlying social or psychological drivers that cause the reasoning of actors. For example, a communication skills course may achieve different outcomes for doctors or nurses. The different reasoning of nurses and doctors relate to dominant social norms about professional roles and hierarchy.

Outcomes

Learning outcomes are the result of the learning mechanism in a particular context.

general enough to be applicable to different scenarios. There is no limit to the number of CMOs that one can develop.

As an education leader, one can collect data to test the proposed learning CMOs. This process is repeated until the middle range theories develop over time based on the findings—that is, the most appropriate way to deliver the learning programme. This process is shown in Fig. 7.1.

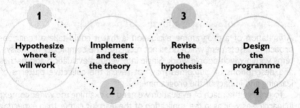

Fig. 7.1 Evaluation of an education programme.
Based on Pawson and Tilley (1997).

How does it work in practice?

There are four steps to take in evaluation of a programme. To illustrate the theory, realist evaluation is used to assess a simulation-based course for nursing students in Box 7.3.

Box 7.3 Steps in evaluation of a programme

Step 1

Formulate a working theory: for example, the simulation course will improve student nurses' confidence and skills before starting work placements

Step 2

Formulate the hypothetical CMO configurations, for example:

First configuration

- *Context*—nursing students who have no practical experience.
- *Mechanism*—providing students with the experience of what it is like to work as a nurse in a setting which is simulated.
- *Outcome*—students have a better understanding of what it is like to work in a clinical setting.

Second configuration

- *Context*—nursing students with no experience of managing a deteriorating patient.
- *Mechanism*—using a simulation dummy, scenarios of various deteriorating patients are acted out.
- *Outcome*—students are better at the practical management of a patient who is deteriorating.

Step 3

Test the theories by gathering data on the CMOs using quantitative and qualitative data collection and analysis. Students participated in focus groups after the course on their experiences and completed questionnaires. The results are analysed.

Step 4

Reveal what worked, for whom, in what circumstances, and why. This will then refine the theory and can be used in future interventions.

Limitations of realist evaluation of programmes

A limitation of a programme evaluation is that it could take a linear approach of assessment which does not recognize the complexity of the systems within which people work. Single intervention evaluation approaches and descriptions of outcomes may not reveal the collective patterns of learning and impact of the programme.

To enlarge the reach of evaluation we need to examine the wider context in learning as well as in the application of the learning rather than expecting single programme outcomes (Box 7.4). Linear cause-and-effect explanations in education evaluation are very difficult, and realistic evaluation may provide a model to understand how people learn.

Box 7.4 Top tips to designing a learning programme

- Learning is complex not linear.
- Use different methods for different contexts.
- Build assessments of learning methods in different contexts to achieve good learning outcomes.

References

Laurillard, D. (2002). *Rethinking University Teaching: A Conversational Framework for the Effective Use of Learning Technologies.* New York: RoutledgeFalmer.

Pawson, R. (2013). *The Science of Realist Evaluation. A Realist Manifesto.* London: Sage.

Pawson, R. and Tilley, N. (1997). *Realistic Evaluation.* Thousand Oaks, CA: SAGE.

Further reading

Weiss, C. (2000). Which links in which theories should we evaluate? *New Directions for Evaluation,* 87, 35–45. https://doi.org/10.1002/ev.1180

Coaching and mentoring in medical education

What are coaching and mentoring?

Coaching and mentoring are development activities that have a key role in the development of leaders, both inside and outside of healthcare systems, although they exist as separate concepts in traditional clinical education.

Why is this important?

Healthcare is rapidly evolving, with new information emerging constantly. Healthcare professionals recognize the need for lifelong learning of advances in clinical care and the importance of staying abreast of best practice. Coaching and mentoring are essential to ensure ongoing development, especially after one ends training.

What is the theory?

Similarities between coaching and mentoring

The key elements are feedback and the action taken to continually improve. Both require a clear commitment and a safe space, both psychologically and practically.

Coaching and mentoring are appropriate at any stage of one's career, regardless of seniority. There is growing evidence on the benefits of being coached or mentored in a more formal way, though either can be informal as well. As there is a need to develop a safe space to work, the benefits include building resilience and reducing stress and anxiety.

Each relies on a transparent and trustworthy relationship between the coach or mentor and the individual receiving the coaching or mentoring, with goals for the interaction that are broad or narrow, depending on the context, which can be re-focused and re-moulded as the relationship progresses.

Differences between coaching and mentoring

Coaching is the process by which an individual is guided towards performance improvement. It is more readily associated with high-performing elites or athletes but has gained recognition within medicine and medical education. Coaching in medical education can be thought of as two types: coaching in the moment (CiM) and coaching over time (CoT) (Table 7.2).

Table 7.2 Coaching in the moment and coaching over time

	Definition	What it involves
CiM	Coaching which takes place between teacher and learner in the clinical environment	Feedback which is based on observations
CoT	Coaching which takes place between teacher and learner outside the clinical environment	Feedback which is based on learner's performance data over time

Mentoring supports or guides career progression, although the 'traditional' definitions have been blurred in that, increasingly, it is the recipient who guides both types of encounters.

Both approaches may vary by individual circumstances, for example, with the amount of information transfer, the nature of the guidance, whether there is a specific requirement for subject knowledge or expertise, the extent to which the encounter is goal-orientated, the level of formality or informality, and the duration of the relationship.

GROW model

The GROW ('Grow, Reality, Options, Will') model is designed to provide a framework of setting the goal of the session, discussing the current reality, exploring the options available, and then setting the actions that need to be taken. An adapted version is shown in Table 7.3.

Table 7.3 Adapted GROW model

Goal	Set a clear goal for what is to be discussed and the outcomes to be achieved
Reality	Check in what is happening now, where are you?
Options	What can you and what will you do? Generate ideas that may or may not work.
Will	What will you do in the next period? Plan for future action

Before one starts, one should define the purpose of the coaching—whether it is for a specific purpose or for mentoring over a longer period. This requires clarity about where you want to be in terms of career.

This starting point may help you lean towards a coach, if you are aware of where you want to be and have clear and specific goals pertaining to this, or a mentor if you feel you would benefit from broader career-related advice and discussion.

For some tips for success, see Box 7.5.

Box 7.5 Tips for success

To select a coach or mentor consider the following
- Clinical subject.
- Inside or outside your current organization.
- Inside or outside your field or profession.
- Medical or non-medical.
- Peer or senior.
- Reverse coaching by a newer member of the team or junior, trusted individual, or new contact.
- Application to or entry into formal coaching or mentoring schemes.

Consider the aims of the relationship
- Skills.
- Projects.
- Careers.
- Problem-solving.
- Brainstorming.
- Resolving conflict.
- Motivation or inspiration.

Consider your requirements for the relationship
- Virtual or in person.
- Short or long duration.
- Fixed or flexible; formal or informal.
- Advice or exploration; career or personal.

Signposting

The Healthcare Leadership Academy (n.d.). *Online Resources.* [online] Available at: https://thehealthcareleadership.academy/ (accessed 3/10/2021).

The NHS (London) Leadership Academy (n.d.). *Online Resources.* [online] Available at: http://www.londonleadershipacademy.nhs.uk/ (accessed 3/10/2021).

Whitmore J. (n.d.). *The Grow Model of Coaching Online Resources.* [online] Available at: https://www.performanceconsultants.com/grow-model (accessed 3/10/2021).

Further reading

Clutterbuck, D. (2008). What's happening in coaching and mentoring? And what is the difference between them? *Development and Learning in Organizations: An International Journal,* 22(4), 8–10. https://doi:10.1108/14777280810886364

Frenk, J., Chen, L., Bhutta, Z.A., et al. (2010). Health professionals for a new century: transforming education to strengthen health systems in an interdependent world. *Lancet,* 376(9756), 1923–1958. doi:10.1016/s0140-6736(10)61854-5

Gallo, A. (2011). Demystifying mentoring. *Harvard Business Review,* 1 February. Available at: https://hbr.org/2011/02/demystifying-mentoring.html (accessed 3/10/2021).

Grant, A.M., Studholme, I., Verma, R., et al. (2017). The impact of leadership coaching in an Australian healthcare setting. *Journal of Health Organization and Management,* 31(2), 237–252. doi:10.1108/jhom-09-2016-0187

Landreville, J., Cheung, W., Frank, J., et al. (2019). A definition for coaching in medical education. *Canadian Medical Education Journal,* 10(4), e109–e110. Available at: https://www.ncbi.nlm.nih.gov/pmc/articles/PMC6892322/ (accessed 3/10/2021).

Le Comte, L. and McClelland, B. (2017). An evaluation of a leadership development coaching and mentoring programme. *Leadership in Health Services,* 30(3), 309–329. doi:10.1108/lhs-07-2016-0030

Sambunjak, D., Straus, S.E. and Marusic, A. (2009). A systematic review of qualitative research on the meaning and characteristics of mentoring in academic medicine. *Journal of General Internal Medicine,* 25(1), 72–78. doi:10.1007/s11606-009-1165-8

Inter-professionalism

What is inter-professionalism?

Inter-professionalism is the act of two or more health professionals collaborating to provide better patient care. This can include patients, families, and communities to deliver care. Inter-professional education is 'when students from two or more professions learn about, from and with each other to enable effective collaboration and improve health outcomes'. The goal of inter-professional education is to prepare healthcare professionals to work together as equal partners, in an integrated system with cohesive practices and common goals.

Why is this important?

Inter-professionalism and the resultant collaborative practice strengthens health systems and improves health outcomes. The increasing clinical complexity has resulted in sub-specialization and the absence of inter-professional collaboration and communication can result in disjointed, fragmented, and duplicative care. Inter-professionalism is required to achieve safe and effective, coordinated, PCC. By working together, the increased demands placed on healthcare providers can be minimized.

During the COVID-19 pandemic, the value of inter-professionalism became paramount to meet the increased demand on clinical services. The new ways of working demonstrated that teams could achieve good outcomes by working with a shared focus, consistent involvement, and good leadership. In the longer term, this can lead to better care at lower cost. Inter-professional education prepares teams to be able to work together under all conditions.

What is the theory?

Inter-professional care represents the democratization of both care delivery and leadership. It requires leaders to possess both professional competency and the ability to nurture team dynamics. Elements of inter-professional collaboration include responsibility, accountability, coordination, communication, cooperation, assertiveness, autonomy, mutual trust, and respect. The collaborative equal partnership achieves the end goal.

The acquisition of good inter-professional practice ideally begins in undergraduate training, and then continues into postgraduate education. Studies have found that introducing interpersonal learning at undergraduate level produces a more positive attitude on working collaboratively' (in students from medicine, nursing, physical therapy, and pharmacy). The development of inter-professional education at each level requires the interaction of the educator and curriculum mechanisms which are listed in Table 7.4.

Once an inter-professional workforce is ready, the mechanisms listed in Table 7.5 are required to develop inter-professional practice.

Interaction between the education system and the professional system leads to a practical concept of inter-professionalism. To achieve inter-professionalism for improved patient outcomes, the interacting systems of education with the learner at the centre, and professional working with the patient at the heart, can be visualized as influenced by the concentric rings of organizational factors surrounding them, within the overall policy and cultural environment.

Table 7.4 Educator mechanisms and curricular mechanisms

Educator mechanisms	Curricular mechanisms
Training of educators	Logistics and scheduling
Champions within the organization	Programme content
Institutional support	Mandatory attendance
Managerial commitment	Shared learning objectives
Learning outcomes to reflect inter-professional goals, incorporation of inter-professional mentorship.	Principles of adult learning
	Contextual learning

Table 7.5 Mechanisms to develop an inter-professional practice

Institutional support mechanisms	Working culture mechanisms	Environmental mechanisms
Governance models	Communication strategies	Built environment facilities
Structured protocols	Conflict resolution policies	Space design to eliminate barriers and hierarchy and facilitate communication and groups
Shared operating resources	Shared decision-making processes	
Personnel policies		
Supportive management practices		

The barriers to achieving inter-professional education and practice are listed in Box 7.6.

Box 7.6 Barriers to inter-professional education and practice

There are several barriers to consider when setting up inter-professional learning:
1. Professional cultures and stereotypes, reinforced by segregated training and socialization, and pre-formed views of professional identities at student level.
2. Established hierarchies, including perceived physician dominance in decision-making.
3. Monopolies over particular knowledge or skills leading to turf wars.
4. Lack of understanding of roles and scope of other professions, including misconceptions.
5. Advocacy for different professions may appear to be at odds with inter-professionalism.
6. Profession-specific accreditation criteria and the absence of inter-professional competencies.
7. Inconsistent terminology—interdisciplinary, multidisciplinary.

These barriers can be addressed by taking a systematic approach to implementing an inter-professional learning programme as shown in Box 7.7.

Box 7.7 Approaches to develop inter-professional education and practice

Teaching factors
- Physical learning environment—location, space is important.
- Temporal learning environment—scheduling when convenient.
- Teach collaborative approaches including exposure to examples of successful and unsuccessful inter-professional working.
- Address beliefs and stereotypes around benefits/challenges of inter-professional working, including helping learners to understand own professional identity and those of others.
- Explore the duties and boundaries of each team role, all applicable to junior as well as faculty and senior staff.

Institutional factors
- Need an institutional vision of inter-professional working (refer to other chapters on achieving change).
- Include champions for the approach and senior buy-in, who may come from any or all of the professions included but are critical to demonstrating effective approaches.

Organizational factors
- Methods for information exchange and capture.
- Administrative support and coordination.
- Restructuring of clinical care into teams to allow inter-professional collaboration.
- Leadership supportive of inter-professional working.
- Practical leadership of inter-professional teams.
- Shared protocols within inter-professional teams.

Cultural factors
- Acknowledgement of the rationale and benefits.
- Managerial and leadership support, enabled by demonstration of benefit and results of collaboration from an early stage.

Environmental factors
- Space to allow inter-professional meetings.
- Technology to support communication.
- Co-location of teams and services to promote collaboration and communication.

How does this work in practice?

An example of how this works in practice is shown in Box 7.8 (based on Partridge et al., 2018). It is important to implement a process co-produced by different team members as equal partners in the inter-professional practice.

For some tips for success, see Box 7.9.

Box 7.8 Case study: preoperative assessment of elderly patients requiring surgery

Background

Concerns about inadequacy of care of vulnerable older patients undergoing surgery with adverse outcomes as a result. Due to the complexity of their physical, mental, and social state, there is a need to optimize physical, psychosocial, and functional well-being before and after surgery in older patients, so as to improve adverse postoperative outcomes, reduce length of stay, and prevent cancellations of surgery.

Intervention

The evidence-based comprehensive geriatric assessment (CGA) is used to identify and address medical, psychosocial, and functional needs, with a clear plan for management and follow-up.

Staff education

Follow-up postoperative review, home visits, and linkage with other services as required.

Team

The team is comprised of a consultant geriatrician, nurse specialist in older people, occupational therapist, physiotherapist, social worker, and administrator.

Actions

Outreach to people receiving care, consultants, and GPs. Development of inter-professional meetings, emergency department liaison, a preassessment clinic incorporating anaesthetist, further education, training, audit, and research.

Outcomes

Reduced medical complications, addressing multidisciplinary issues in a timely manner, and decreased length of stay.

Box 7.9 Tips for success

Ideas to explore in the formation of effective inter-professional working

- Formation of groups to deliver inter-professional team-based care (care delivered by intentionally created groups with a collective identity and shared responsibility for a patient group (see 'Signposting'), e.g. rapid response team, primary care team, operating theatre team).
- Formation of learning or planning groups outside the traditional auspices of care (e.g. paediatric, school and primary care meetings; public health and hospital clinician joint meetings).
- Schwartz rounds to share experiences.
- Inter-professional innovation teams, competitions, and initiatives.
- Inter-professional cross-disciplinary further education (e.g. leadership training, quality improvement).
- Co-location of care (e.g. medical home concept, such as co-location of antenatal and substance abuse treatment for women, co-location of social workers and primary care).

Ideas for effective inter-professional learning

- Case-based or journal club-style inter-professional group learning.
- Inter-professional team simulation.
- The role of inter-professional feedback in the form of assessments, multisource feedback.
- Inter-professional coaching and mentorship.
- Inter-professional volunteering opportunities.

Signposting

Interprofessional Education Collaborative (2011). *Core Competencies for Interprofessional Collaborative Practice.* Washington, DC: Interprofessional Education Collaborative. Available at: https://www.aacom.org/docs/default-source/insideome/ccrpt05-10-11.pdf?sfvrsn=77937f97_2 (accessed 3/10/2021).

Reference

Partridge, J., Sbai, M., and Dhesi, J. (2018). Proactive care of older people undergoing surgery. *Aging Clinical and Experimental Research*, 30(3), 253–257. doi:10.1007/s40520-017-0879-4

Further reading

Alruwaili, A., Mumenah, N., Alharthy, N., et al. (2020). Students' readiness for and perception of interprofessional learning: a cross-sectional study. *BMC Medical Education*, 20(1). doi:10.1186/s12909-020-02325-9

D'Amour, D. and Oandasan, I. (2005). Interprofessionality as the field of interprofessional practice and interprofessional education: an emerging concept. *Journal of Interprofessional Care*, 19(Suppl 1), 8–20. doi:10.1080/13561820500081604

Global Forum on Innovation in Health Professional Education Board on Global Health National Academies of Sciences, Engineering, and Medicine (2013). *Interprofessional Education for Collaboration: Learning How to Improve Health from Interprofessional Models Across the Continuum of Education to Practice: Workshop Summary.* Washington, DC: National Academies Press. Available at: https://www.nap.edu/read/13486/chapter/1#ii (accessed 3/10/2021).

Woltenberg, L., Aulisio, M., Erlandson, E., et al. (2019). Interprofessional leadership development for health professions learners: a program and outcomes review. *Education in the Health Professions*, 2(1), 19. doi:10.4103/ehp.ehp_1_19

World Health Organization (2013). *Interprofessional Collaborative Practice in Primary Health Care: Nursing and Midwifery Perspectives.* [online] World Health Organization. Available at: https://apps.who.int/iris/handle/10665/120098

Career transitions

Why is this important?

A clinical career consists of different stages, starting in medical school, each with their own demands. During the training years, trainees are assessed by a mixture of methods, including examinations for knowledge and competency-based assessments, as well as interviews and team-based interactions. The different phases of training culminate in the trainee becoming an independent practitioner, either as a consultant or as a GP, with increased responsibility, accountability, and financial rewards, as well as the ability to influence and contribute to change. Embracing each new level of seniority can be difficult, due to the added pressures of time and responsibility.

Each career stage transition can be thought of as a change in one's level of mastery, or expertise. Learning can be defined as a permanent change in one's capability to perform a skill. Ericsson et al. (2007) advocate an apprenticeship and deliberate practice-based path to expertise and theorize that one requires 10,000 hours of deliberate practice to achieve 'expertise'. While it is debatable whether clinical medicine is best modelled on an 'apprenticeship' model of learning or not, each career transition results in the attainment of new competencies.

What is the theory?

Vygotsky (1986) proposed the importance of the 'zone of proximal development' (ZPD) as a situation where an individual can build on existing skills with scaffolded learning support to be able to develop new skills, initially outside of their expertise. This is represented in Fig. 7.2.

If we think about this being the conclusion of one stage of training and a career transition into another, it is evident that this is also a potentially dangerous time where processes, such as clinical supervision, reflective practice, and coaching/mentoring move towards autonomy, require support to empower the trainee to work at the maxims of the ZPD.

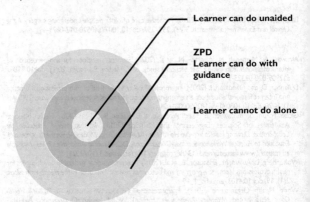

Learner can do unaided

ZPD
Learner can do with guidance

Learner cannot do alone

Fig. 7.2 The zone of proximal development (ZPD).

This must be recognized by the trainee and the educational supervisor/coach/mentor and planned for appropriately.

Continuing professional development

Miller (1990) proposed the prism of clinical competence which has underpinned the pedagogical basis of workplace-based assessments (WPBAs). These are an integral part of a competency-based system. There are four stages from knowledge assessment to the assessment of the application of that knowledge in the workplace. The key components of Miller's prism are shown in Table 7.6.

Table 7.6 Levels of assessment

Level	Focus of assessment	How assessed
Know	Assess knowledge that has been gained in the learning	Multiple choice questions
How	Assess application knowledge and its integration into action. Integrate and interpret the information gathered into understanding how it can be applied	Case studies, reflections, and essays in which the knowledge must be applied
Show	Is able to demonstrate the application of the knowledge into action	Simulation, objective structured clinical examination (OSCE)
Does	The knowledge is applied in practice to demonstrate it has been integrated into active application	Observation in the workplace to demonstrate performance

An effective WPBA can provide valuable and directed feedback that can support the learner. This in turn drives CPD. The learning benefit is enhanced when the feedback is specific. Experiential learning is beneficial, and learning is optimized when practice and feedback are combined and WPBA is part of the longitudinal monitoring of trainees. Miller proposed a journey from knowing to doing—one moves from knowledge to skills and application of the knowledge.

Reflective practice

The Academy of Medical Educators emphasizes the importance of reflective practice as underpinning its core values and alludes to its potential use in CPD. CPD is an integral part of appraisals (see Appraisal and personal development plans, p. 37) with appraisees having to formulate a career development plan and demonstrate the steps that they have taken to achieve the set outcomes. To achieve this, the appraisee needs to reflect on skills, attitudes, and behaviours.

The GMC CPD guidance for doctors identifies the principles of reflective practice which are a key element of education (Box 7.10). Clinical leaders facilitate reflection as a central principle of learning.

Box 7.10 General Medical Council principles for continuing professional development

Principles of continuing professional development

The purpose of CPD is to help improve the safety and quality of care provided for patients and the public.

Responsibility for personal learning

You are responsible for identifying your CPD needs, planning how those needs should be addressed, and undertaking CPD that will support your professional development and practice.

Reflection

Good Medical Practice requires you to reflect regularly on your standards of medical practice.

Scope of practice

You must remain competent and up to date in all areas of your practice. Your CPD activities should aim to maintain and improve the standards of your own practice and those of any teams in which you work.

Identification of needs

Your CPD activities should be shaped by assessments of both your professional needs and the needs of the service and the people who use it.

Outcomes

You must reflect on what you have learnt through your CPD and record any impact (or expected future impact) on your performance and practice.

Signposting

Academy of Medical Educators (2021). *Professional Standards*, 4th ed. London: Academy of Medical Educators. Available at: https://www.medicaleducators.org/write/MediaManager/Documents/AoME_Professional_Standards_4th_edition_1.0_(web_full_single_page_spreads).pdf (accessed 3/10/2021).

References

Ericsson, K.A., Prietula, M.J., and Cokely, E.T. (2007). The making of an expert. *Harvard Business Review*, July–Aug. Available at: https://hbr.org/2007/07/the-making-of-an-expert (accessed 3/10/2021).

Miller, G.E. (1990). The assessment of clinical skills/competence/performance. *Academic Medicine*, 65(9), S63–S67. doi:10.1097/00001888-199009000-00045

Vygotsky, L.S. (1986). The development of scientific concepts in childhood. In: A. Kozulin A (ed) *Thought and Language* (pp. 146–209). Cambridge, MA: MIT Press.

Further reading

General Medical Council (2012). *Guidance on Continuing Professional Development for Doctors*. London: General Medical Council. Available at: https://www.gmc-uk.org/-/media/documents/cpd-guidance-for-all-doctors-0316_pdf-56438625.pdf (accessed 3/10/2021).

Hesketh, E.A., Bagnall, G., Buckley, E.G., et al. (2001). A framework for developing excellence as a clinical educator. *Medical Education*, 35(6), 555–564. doi:10.1046/j.1365-2923.2001.00920.x

Rolfe, I.E. and Sanson-Fisher, R.W. (2002). Translating learning principles into practice: a new strategy for learning clinical skills. *Medical Education*, 36(4), 345–352. doi:10.1046/j.1365-2923.2002.01170.x

Effective feedback for learning

What is effective feedback for learning?

Learning and feedback are closely coupled. Feedback is a set of practices over time, with the dual intention to improve immediate work and future work. Receptivity to feedback is embedded within conditions for its uptake, such as perceived relevance to the learner, motivation, trust of the source and opportunities for negotiated goals.

Feedback refers to the process of obtaining information which enables change through adjustment or calibration of efforts to bring a person (or group) closer to a well-defined goal. It is an active two-way engagement between educator and learner and/or peers and learner(s) (see Chapter 2 for further skills).

Why is it important?

Feedback is important for learning because people want to know how to improve. The vital role that feedback plays in assisting learners to improve their performance has been recognized from the beginnings of behavioural science. Receiving feedback enables learners to close a critical gap between the current performance and a desired level (standard) of performance. The purpose of feedback is to reduce the gap.

Length of time in a profession is not a guarantee of performance and the drop off effect (i.e. deterioration in performance with increasing time in the role) is well researched. Elite performers rely on high-calibre coaches to provide a continuing critique. Implicit is an idea of continual learning. While practising an activity allows you to shift control from a conscious to an automatic function, automaticity pegs your skill at a given level. Incremental improvement will come from external feedback and the effort to apply this in future tasks.

In healthcare systems, learning through feedback is key to safety. The growing internationalization of the healthcare workforce poses cultural challenges to educators and learners. Attention should be given to enabling staff to participate effectively in the feedback conversation and acquire skills in both 'seeking' and giving 'feedback'.

What is the theory?

Feedback has roots in biology which involves the control of a system by re-inserting into the system the results of its performance (e.g. homeostasis). The difference in the application of this idea to education and learning is that the learner can choose to accept or reject the feedback. Information does not act automatically, as it must be processed by learners who must decide whether to act on it to achieve a changed 'output'. Therefore, for feedback to be effective we must move beyond how to deliver it: we must include what happens prior to educator inputs. Feedback in education should not be unsolicited or one way, but must engage the learner to be successful. Learners are more likely to increase effort when the intended goal is clear, when high commitment is secured for it, and when belief in eventual success is high (Fig. 7.3).

Implicit in the feedback conversation is an idea of social modelling. Social modelling allows the learner (or learners) an opportunity to discuss and observe the skills possessed or displayed by a competent individual. We are

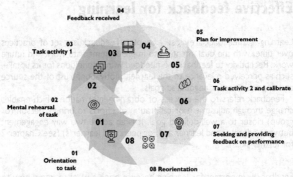

Fig. 7.3 Feedforward and feedback.

biologically hardwired to acquire considerable knowledge through this kind of 'vicarious' learning. Furthermore, when observing performers in your domain, you can evaluate critical aspects not seen by others. Similarly, feedback also cues educators to deficiencies within their education and training programme.

Challenges in healthcare

The complexities of work-based learning environments challenge our ability to provide feedback. Continuing learning in work requires our staff to take their own initiatives to seek and utilize feedback—to plan and manage their performance. Educational and training programmes across healthcare should include components to build capacity to seek and deliver feedback (Box 7.11). This involves the management of the social and cultural dimensions of the clinical workplace.

Activities involving collective mental rehearsal and seeking feedback are ways of hugely multiplying opportunities to promote learning and cultural literacy. But importantly, they are also ways of belonging to a community. Barriers that exist to providing good feedback include a fear of upsetting others or damaging the relationship with them and this is a common issue in healthcare settings.

Box 7.11 Components of feedback

Key components

Feedback involves:
- criterion (relative to a standard)
- clarification of understandings or misconceptions
- developing judgement, criticism, and evaluation
- opportunities to develop feedback seeking/giving skills
- confirmation of good practice
- correction (focus on pros and cons)
- comments on how to proceed in future.

Feedback principles

To make feedback more effective, educators should:
- focus on how feedback is received rather than how it is delivered
- frame feedback in terms of what learners do (and will do)
- negotiate with learners the goals of feedback (including exploration of learner priorities)
- make the criteria for success transparent and explicit (before the task)
- prime performance through collective mental rehearsal
- engage learners at or just above their current level of functioning
- create psychological safety in the environment so that it is open to errors and to disconfirmation
- facilitate peer feedback practices as a valuable platform for continuous learning in groups.

Further reading

Boud, D. and Molloy, E. (2013). *Feedback in Higher and Professional Education*. London: Routledge.

Foster-Collins, H., Conn, R., Dornan, T., et al. (2021). The problem with feedback. *MedEdPublish*, 10, 128. https://doi.org/10.15694/mep.2021.000128.1

Hattie, J. and Yates, G. (2013). *Visible Learning and the Science of How we Learn*. London: Routledge.

Kluger, A.N. and Van Dijk, D. (2010). Feedback, the various tasks of the doctor, and the feedforward alternative. *Medical Education*, 44(12), 1166–1174. doi:10.1111/j.1365-2923.2010.03849.x

Ley, T., Kisielewska, J., Collett, T., et al. (2019). Improving communication for learning with students: expectations, feedback and feedforward. *MedEdPublish*, 8, 14. doi:10.15694/mep.2019.000014.1

Patient safety and human factors learning

What is learning for patient safety?

In Chapter 3, leadership for patient safety was discussed and the importance of protecting the people who receive care and ensuring the safety of those who deliver care was emphasized. The achievement of safe care learning requires proactive learning programmes.

Why is this important?

The magnitude of harm is an enormous public health issue. The need for a robust culture of openness, probity, and for blame-free management of incidents of harm, as well as a proactive approach to the prevention of such harm, requires patient safety and its management to be addressed in medical education at each level. The Berwick report on Mid-Staffordshire NHS Foundation Trust called for clinicians to undertake lifelong learning to achieve the competencies required to be safe.

The facilitation of safe clinical systems is dependent on the development of clinical staff who understand the theories and the methods of patient safety. This includes:

- teaching an approach to safety
- understanding the theories of incident investigation, human factors, systems thinking, reliability, and resilience
- developing a culture of responsibility without blame and an approach to understanding the systems surrounding patients and doctors which lead to error.

Future medical curricula will require the development of leaders who are well versed in the theories and methods of patient safety. This includes understanding human factors and ergonomics, clinical risk management and incident investigation, reliability theory, and resilience learning and application to daily practice.

Why is patient safety important for learning?

To be safe, clinicians need to take the following actions:

1. *Be preoccupied with potential failure* by acknowledging and planning for the possibility of failure due to the high-risk, error-prone nature of their activities.
2. *Commit to resilience* by proactively seeking out unexpected threats and contain them before they cause harm.
3. *Be sensitive to operations* paying close attention to the issues facing workers on the frontline.
4. *Develop a culture of safety* in which individuals feel comfortable drawing attention to potential hazards or actual failures without fear of criticism from others—that is, develop psychological safety.

Why is learning about resilience important?

The theory is that human performance can only be understood by studying how to respond to a constantly changing environment and changing circumstances. This approach implies that we need to include the study of systems and the development of resilience in a learning system as a central part of how we teach patient safety.

How does this work in practice?

Patient safety must be included in all levels of training and learning for trainees and clinicians. As leaders, we need to develop programmes in which we learn from what went wrong—using tools such as RCA, as well as from what goes right—that is, how we adapt to changing circumstances and constantly adapt to avoid harm (Box 7.12). This is a feature of working in complex adaptive systems.

> **Box 7.12 Top tips for teaching and learning patient safety**
>
> - Identify the learning objectives for your audience.
> - Ascertain what is included in the existing curriculum, whether at formal course or the departmental teaching programme.
> - Build into the existing elements of the curriculum in preference to viewing safety as a new subject to teach. Safety should complement and coordinate with existing teaching material at all levels since it is common to all areas of clinical practice and each specialty and clinical area has its own unique patient safety challenges.
> - Consider the capacity of teaching colleagues to address areas of patient safety.
> - Identify like-minded colleagues or champions to collaborate and start the process. Initial education for other colleagues may be necessary in the form of reading and workshops. This approach is overall ideally inter-professional, since safety is not solely a medical concern.
> - Patient safety teaching is best delivered in the workplace or environment to which it is relevant and case examples are best if relevant to the specialty or clinical area in question. Context, realism, the use of practical examples, the ability to explore or practise safely (e.g. through simulation) a culture of support and not criticism are all key to effective learning in patient safety.
> - Role modelling and living expected behaviours helps to demonstrate an approach to safety and openness centred around avoidance of hierarchies, blame, and shame, accepting of fallibility, and promotion of teamwork.
> - Include patient stories in the teaching.
> - Learn from past incidents of what worked well and what did not.
> - Establish a journal club for review of latest papers.
> - Learn from other industries and other health facilities and teams.
> - Use simulation to practise and learn.
> - Maximize the potential learning in morbidity/mortality meetings and serious untoward event analyses.
> - Mentoring and role modelling around patient safety behaviours.

Signposting

Berwick, D.M. (2013). *A promise to Learn – A Commitment to Act: Improving the Safety of Patients in England*. London: The Stationary Office. Available at: https://www.gov.uk/government/uploads/system/uploads/attachment_data/file/226703/Berwick_Report.pdf (accessed 3/10/2021).

Further reading

Holden, R.J., Carayon, P., Gurses, A.P., et al. (2013). SEIPS 2.0: a human factors framework for studying and improving the work of healthcare professionals and patients. *Ergonomics*, 56(11), 1669–1686. doi:10.1080/00140139.2013.838643

Sujan, M.A., Furniss, D., Anderson, J., et al. (2019). Resilient health care as the basis for teaching patient safety—a safety-II critique of the World Health Organization patient safety curriculum. *Safety Science*, 118, 15–21. doi:10.1016/j.ssci.2019.04.046

Vosper, H., Hignett, S., and Bowie, P. (2017). Twelve tips for embedding human factors and ergonomics principles in healthcare education. *Medical Teacher*, 40(4), 357–363. doi:10.1080/0142159x.2017.1387240

Introduction to simulation

What is simulation?

Simulation is any education activity using aides to replicate a clinical scenario. It often involves the use of specially programmed mannequins, as well as the use of simulation involving actors allowing relatively realistic exposure to challenging clinical scenarios, while minimizing risk to patients and staff. It offers the opportunity to improve clinical and interpersonal skills through rehearsal and practice.

Why is it important?

The benefits of simulation are wide ranging. Often, the effectiveness of the educational debrief after a simulated scenario can be equally useful to the learner as the simulated scenario in terms of embedding learning. It is important to note that a fair proportion of the published research into simulation has focused on its use as an assessment tool rather than a training method, though in recent years this has changed considerably.

As a modality, simulation offers great opportunities for developing our understanding of learning, because it is consistent with very different ways of conceptualizing learning. As such, simulation training proves to be relevant and accessible to a wide variety of staff, from different professions and disciplines, with different preferred learning styles. Therefore, simulation as a modality serves to enhance the learning of the participant, utilizing the participant's preferred learning style as a 'lens'.

Simulation serves to be a powerful modality of learning in an interprofessional context, where participants derive learning from different parts of the simulated scenario. While some learn from the experiential feel of being immersed in the simulation itself, others derive more learning from the post-simulation debrief. This demonstrates a preference for a specific learning typology, as advocated by Honey and Mumford (1992), which in turn is extrapolated from Kolb's experiential learning cycle (Fig. 7.4). It states that people indicate a preference for being reflectors, theorists, pragmatists, and activists as they engage in various parts of an experiential learning cycle.

Simulation lends itself very well to Kolb's initial cycle, as different parts of the simulation session, such as a concrete experience in the simulation immersion, as well as observation and reflection in the debrief, map nicely onto the cycle.

Simulation has tended to be used more by anaesthetic and surgical specialties. This is changing, with increasingly powerful use of simulation in several different settings and subject areas, such as mental health, including providing innovative training to support healthcare workers in the management of patients with comorbidities.

Crucially, as care is integrated across traditionally distinct subject domains (e.g. mental healthcare and physical healthcare) and different environments (primary and secondary care), it is apparent that as clinical services develop in this manner, education and training should as well. This encourages the routine embedding of specific simulation-based training programmes into curriculums, and allows healthcare practitioners to develop their understanding of human factors and relevant 'non-technical skills.

Simulation benefits staff and patients by allowing staff to create mistakes in a safe and supportive environment, away from the patient. Simulation

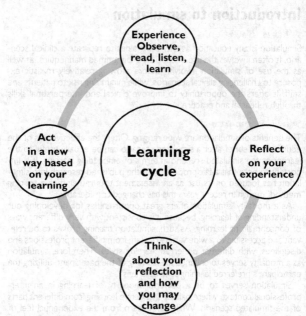

Fig. 7.4 Adapted Kolb experiential learning cycle.

as a modality is used in different ways by different safety critical industries; however, in healthcare it is an effective modality bridging both education and training, and the world of quality improvement.

Currently, there are standards for simulation-based education in healthcare in the UK, set by the Association for Simulated Practice in Healthcare. Simulation-based training is provided by several NHS and private providers. Increasingly, *in situ* simulation is being used to provide training to staff within the clinical environment using mobile equipment as well as remote and VR/AR technologies which saw a marked rise in use during the Covid-19 pandemic.

What is the theory?

There are several different models of simulation, some of which aim to concentrate on driving learning by encouraging discussion about human factors ergonomics.

- McGaghie et al. (2010) reviewed published simulation research and discussed 12 best-practice factors that contribute to effective simulation and debriefing of the simulated scenarios. The review describes the importance of feedback in medicine to debriefing simulation.
- Salas et al. (2008) provide a list of best-practice tips for debriefing simulation. They indicate that 'the delay between task performance and feedback' should be shortened. This checklist of best practice emphasizes the importance of 'educating team leaders in the art and

science of debrief'. However, there is a limited evidence base as to how to translate this into practice.

- Rudolph et al. (2008) advocate a four-step model of debriefing feedback based around keeping the discussion concerned with addressing a 'gap' from the predetermined objectives and basically describing these, providing feedback on these, investigating the basis for these, and then addressing how to close the gap. The authors would argue that by its very definition, simulation is, at its core, an expression of experiential learning.

- Kolb's six propositions of experiential learning theory which are all applicable to simulation. Given that simulation often gives rise to learning and that learning is a 'process whereby knowledge is created through the transformation of experience', applying predetermined objectives and identifying 'gaps' in simulation reduces the validity of any transformative experience. There are no 'right outcomes' in simulation that are not assessment driven. Different outcomes prevail on different occasions and have a multitude of interconnected contributing factors.

Overall whilst simulation is not a panacea, its effective uses involves successful 'pre' and 'de' briefing, consideration to the role of human factors, careful learning needs analysis and evaluation metrics that have clinical 'teeth' and ultimately improve patient care. (Snelgrove and Fernando, 2018).

Signposting

Association for Simulated Practice in Healthcare (2017). *Standards for Simulation-based Education*. Lichfield: Association for Simulated Practice in Healthcare. Available at: http://aspih.org.uk/wp-content/uploads/2017/07/standards-framework.pdf (accessed 3/10/2021).

Simulation in Healthcare. https://journals.lww.com/simulationinhealthcare/pages/default.aspx (accessed 20/07/2022).

References

Honey, P. and Mumford, A. (1992). *The Manual of Learning Styles*. Maidenhead: Ardingly House.

Kolb, A.Y. and Kolb, D.A. (2017). Learning styles and learning spaces: enhancing experiential learning in higher education. *Academy of Management Learning & Education*, 4(2), 193–212. doi:10.5465/amle.2005.17268566

McGaghie, W.C., Issenberg, S.B., Petrusa, E.R., et al. (2010). A critical review of simulation-based medical education research: 2003–2009. *Medical Education*, 44(1), 50–63. doi:10.1111/j.1365-2923.2009.03547.x

Rudolph, J.W., Simon, R., Raemer, D.B., et al. (2008). Debriefing as formative assessment: closing performance gaps in medical education. *Academic Emergency Medicine*, 15(11), 1010–1016. doi:10.1111/j.1553-2712.2008.00248.x

Salas, E., Klein, C., King, H., et al. (2008). Debriefing medical teams: 12 evidence-based best practices and tips. *The Joint Commission Journal on Quality and Patient Safety*, 34(9), 518–527. doi:10.1016/s1553-7250(08)34066-5

Snelgrove, H. and Fernando, A., (2018). Practising forethought: the role of mental simulation. BMJ Simulation & Technology Enhanced Learning, 4(2), 45.

Further reading

Attoe, C., Kowalski, C., Fernando, A., et al. (2016). Integrating mental health simulation into routine health-care education. *Lancet Psychiatry*, 3(8), 702–703. doi:10.1016/s2215-0366(16)30100-6

Index

For the benefit of digital users, indexed terms that span two pages (e.g., 52–53) may, on occasion, appear on only one of those pages.

Tables, figures, and boxes are indicated by *t*, *f*, and *b* following the page number